Ski Hunter

Midlife and Older LGBT Adults
Knowledge and Affirmative Practice for the Social Services

D0162454

More pre-publication
REVIEWS, COMMENTARIES, EVALUATIONS . . .

"This book is an incredibly rich resource for social workers and other social service workers as well as the general public. It is solidly research-based and filled with valuable information within a historical perspective. The Introduction alone is worth the price of the book! The book provides a comprehensive summary and critique of the studies that have been done on midlife and older LGBT persons. It also provides a powerful comparative account of the historical contexts in which older cohorts and midlife cohorts experienced life and the tremendous impacts of Stonewall and the HIV/AIDS crisis. This book should be particularly useful for helping professionals who wish to become more culturally competent in providing services to older GLBT clients."

Dorothy Van Soest, DSW, MSW
Dean and Professor,
University of Washington
School of Social Work

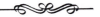

"Dr. Hunter has given social welfare practitioners and those interested in LGBT aging an interesting, extremely well-documented book that is easy to read and not afraid to challenge stereotypes. For anyone looking for information especially related to the challenges and practice issues facing midlife and older lesbian and gay populations, this book is a must buy. Social practitioners and educators who have been previously unable to find an excellent reference related to LGBT aging need look no further—here it is."

Carol T. Tully, PhD
Professor of Social Work,
University of Louisville

"Ski Hunter's book, *Midlife and Older LGBT Adults: Knowledge and Affirmative Practice for the Social Services,* makes an important contribution to the literature in both LGBT studies and gerontology. A strength of the book is its comprehensive review of the existing research in a field that has grown considerably in recent years. The list of references is impressive and useful to any scholar interested in this topic area. Moreover, the book will be useful to practitioners new to the field of LGBT aging. The information is accessible and covers many of the key issues with which practitioners need to be familiar for affirmative practice with this population. Some chapters focus particularly on practice considerations in working with midlife and older LGBT persons—as opposed to LGBT individuals in general—and thus make a unique contribution to the existing practice literature on working with the LGBT population. The author has done an admirable job of including content on bisexual and transgender individuals throughout the book—which is difficult given the limited research on these subpopulations. The attention to racial, ethnic, geographic, and economic diversity throughout the volume makes the content more widely applicable than it would be if the diversity within the LGBT population were ignored.

Sandra S. Butler, PhD, MSW
Associate Professor and Interim Director,
School of Social Work,
University of Maine

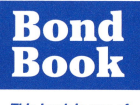

Midlife and Older LGBT Adults
Knowledge and Affirmative Practice for the Social Services

THE HAWORTH PRESS
Titles of Related Interest

Gay Midlife and Maturity: Crises, Opportunities, and Fulfillment edited by John Alan Lee

Gay and Gray: The Older Homosexual Man, Second Edition by Raymond M. Berger

Midlife Lesbian Relationships: Friends, Lovers, Children, and Parents edited by Marcy R. Adelman

Gay Men at Midlife: Age Before Beauty edited by Alan L. Ellis

Housing Choices and Well-Being of Older Adults: Proper Fit edited by Leon A. Pastalan and Benyamin Schwarz

Midlife and Aging in Gay America: Proceedings of the SAGE Conference 2000 edited by Douglas C. Kimmel and Dawn Lundy Martin

Midlife and Older Adults and HIV: Implications for Social Service Research, Practice, and Policy edited by Cynthia Cannon Poindexter and Sharon M. Keigher

Reeling in the Years: Gay Men's Perspectives on Age and Ageism by Tim Bergling

Whistling Women: A Study of the Lives of Older Lesbian Women by Cheryl Claasen

Lives of Lesbian Elders: Looking Back, Looking Forward by D. Merilee Clunis, Karen I. Fredriksen-Goldsen, Pat A. Freeman, and Nancy Nystrom

Dealing with the Psychological and Spiritual Aspects of Menopause: Finding Hope in the Midlife by Dana E. King, Melissa H. Hunter, and Jerri R. Harris

Midlife and Older LGBT Adults
Knowledge and Affirmative Practice for the Social Services

Ski Hunter

The Haworth Press®
New York • London • Oxford

For more information on this book or to order, visit
http://www.haworthpress.com/store/product.asp?sku=5289

or call 1-800-HAWORTH (800-429-6784) in the United States and Canada
or (607) 722-5857 outside the United States and Canada

or contact orders@HaworthPress.com

The Haworth Press, Inc., 10 Alice Street, Binghamton, NY 13904-1580.

Cover design by Marylouise E. Doyle.

Library of Congress Cataloging-in-Publication Data

Hunter, Ski
    Midlife and older LGBT adults : knowledge and affirmative practice for the social services / Ski Hunter.
      p. cm.
    Includes bibliographical references and index.
    ISBN: 0-7890-1835-7 (hard : alk. paper) — ISBN: 0-7890-1836-5 (soft : alk. paper)
    1. Middle aged gays. 2. Older gays. 3. Transsexuals. 4. Social work with gays. 5. Aging. I. Title.

HQ75.15.H86 2005
306.76'6'0844—dc22

2004012742

To Andrea
who delights me with her intellect, intensity, depth,
and in every other way

ABOUT THE AUTHOR

Ski Hunter, PhD, MSW, is a professor at the School of Social Work, University of Texas at Arlington. Among the courses she teaches is a course on LGBT issues. She has presented numerous workshops on this topic. Besides two books on midlife, she was the lead author of *Lesbian, Gay, and Bisexual Youths and Adults* published in 1998, co-author of *Lesbian, Gay, Bisexual, and Transgender Issues in Social Work* published in 2001, and lead author of *Affirmative Practice: Understanding and Working with Gay, Bisexual, and Transgender Persons.*

CONTENTS

PART II: LIFE ARENAS

PART III: POSITIVES VERSUS DOWNTURNS

PART IV: PRACTICE WITH MIDLIFE AND OLDER LGBT PERSONS

Acknowledgments

I wish to acknowledge and thank my friend and former book editor, Steph Selice. She has supported my writing and many other things in my life. And I acknowledge all LGBTI persons who helped pave the way for more openness, connections with one another, and rights.

Introduction

This book examines the context in which midlife and older LGBT persons live and details some of the issues they may need to cope with or overcome. It will lead the reader, whether LGBT (lesbian, gay, bisexual, transgender) person, general reader, teacher, undergraduate or graduate student, or practitioner, through many life contexts of midlife and older LGBT persons. Part I addresses concepts, sexual identities, and terminology (Chapter 1) and coming out and disclosure (Chapter 2). Part II addresses life arenas such as education, work, and community participation (Chapter 3) and couples and other family links (Chapter 4). Part III addresses positives in the lives of midlife and older gay persons (Chapter 5) and transitions and downturns of aging (Chapter 6). Part IV addresses the changes in diagnostics, treatments, and human services (Chapter 7); an overview of practice with midlife and older lesbian and gay persons (Chapter 8); practice issues regarding coming out and disclosure (Chapter 9); practice issues regarding couples and family (Chapter 10); and using groups and community practice with older lesbian and gay persons (Chapter 11). What follows in this chapter is a review of studies done on midlife and older LGBT persons, estimates of the number of this population, when these stages of life occur, and the historical context in which midlife and older LGBT persons were raised.

THE STUDIES

The study of lesbian and gay persons has increased during the past twenty-five years or so (Herdt, 1997; Hostetler & Herdt, 1998). Much of the scholarship has been focused on the developmental processes involved in coming out to oneself as lesbian or gay and disclosing this information to others. Typically, coming out now happens during adolescence and disclosures in late adolescence or early adulthood. Therefore, most of the study on these processes focuses on groups of young persons. Less study has been devoted to these developmental processes across the years of adulthood (Cohler & Boxer, 1984) or to other developmental issues that may be confronted in middle and late adulthood.

Other than research on the "psychopathology" of gay persons, research on any topics in the lives of midlife and older lesbian and gay persons was largely nonexistent until the 1970s (Morin, 1977). A few studies were done on mostly older gay persons (e.g., Berger, 1980, 1982/1996, 1984; Francher & Henkin, 1973; Gray & Dressel, 1985; J. Kelly, 1977; Kimmel, 1977, 1978, 1979, 1979/1980; Lee, 1987; M. S. Weinberg, 1970; M. S. Weinberg & Williams, 1974). Everyone in the samples was usually labeled as older, although some of the studies included men in the midlife age range. The samples are limited in generalizations as they were usually small in number, and the participants were largely white, well educated, urban, upper middle class, and participated in the gay community through friendship networks, bars, or support organizations (Wahler & Gabbay, 1997; L. M. Woolf, 2002).

Documentation of the experiences of midlife and older lesbians began about a decade later (e.g., Adelman, 1986; Almvig, 1982; Copper, 1988; Friend, 1987; Kehoe, 1986, 1989; Kirkpatrick, 1989a, 1989b; MacDonald & Rich, 1983; Raphael & Robinson, 1980; Woodman, 1987). The most extensive data to date on midlife lesbians came from a small set of reports primarily produced in the 1990s (e.g., Bradford & Ryan, 1991; Bridges & Croteau, 1994; Charbonneau & Lander, 1991; Cole & Rothblum, 1991; Fertitta, 1984; Kirkpatrick, 1989a, 1989b; Lander & Charbonneau, 1990; Sang, 1987, 1990, 1991, 1992a, 1992b, 1993; Warshow, 1991; Wyers, 1987). However, these reports are also limited in generalizations as the participants were mainly white, professional, and middle to upper middle class.

The initials LGB or LGBT are used frequently in this book; this does not imply that material on these groups of persons is available in any equivalent way. Far more material is currently available on lesbian and gay persons. In addition, for some topics data exist on midlife persons but not on older persons; for other topics the situation is reversed. Whereas the midlife data focus mostly on lesbians, the data on the older cohort focus mostly on gay persons. Few studies include persons clearly designated to be over age sixty, over age eighty-five, or among the oldest-old. Sometimes the plural "LGBT populations" is used to infer that these populations or communities are diverse or that there are various LGBT communities and often there are important differences among them (L. M. Woolf, 2002). However, little research has been done on midlife and older LGBT persons who are members of various racial or ethic groups (Cahill, South, & Spade, 2000), or diverse in other ways such as social class, the degree their identities are central to their self-definition, their level of affiliation with other LGBT persons, or their rejection or acceptance of societal stereotypes and prejudice about their sexual identities (Meyer, 2001).

Whereas lesbian, gay, and bisexual are sexual identities that often indicate sexual orientations, transgender and intersex are identities that do not represent sexual orientations. Transgender and intersex persons experience the full range of sexual attractions, sexual orientations, and sexual identities. Whatever the differences, all persons under the LGBT label contend with the common issues of stigma, prejudice, discrimination, harassment, and violence. LGBT persons are subject to legal discrimination in housing, employment, and basic civil rights. Across the United States coalitions of LGBT communities recognize common goals of sexual freedom and sex-gender expression. For intersex persons, a major goal is freedom from surgical decisions soon after birth. LGBTI persons also experience common issues such as disclosure of identity information. There is no literature on the midlife and older experiences of transgender and intersex persons, and it is almost nonexistent on bisexual persons. For example, for transgender persons, there are no answers to questions such as the following: What are the effects of long-term use of hormones? What happens when a transgender person enters a long-term care placement? What kind of resources does the transgender community provide for older transgender persons? (Shankle, Maxwell, Katzman, & Landers, 2003).

NUMBERS OF MIDLIFE AND OLDER LGBT PERSONS

No accurate data currently exist for the midlife and older LGBT population in the United States, although there are estimates for these groups. For example, about 1 million gay persons are over the age of forty (Berger & Kelly, 2001). An estimated range of LGB persons over the age of sixty is between 1.75 to 3.5 million (S. Jacobson & Grossman, 1996). Over the past several decades, the number of persons over the age of sixty-five in the general population has increased twice as fast as the rest of the population. The population of older LGB persons is also growing. Cahill et al. (2000) estimated that 1 to 3 million Americans over age sixty-five is LGBT, based on an estimated range of 3 to 8 percent of the overall population of older persons. As is true for the overall older population, the number and proportion of older LGBT persons will increase considerably over the next few decades. By 2030, one in five Americans will be sixty-five or older and about 4 million of this group will be LGBT (Cahill et al., 2000). Again, these figures are only estimates but they are the best figures available until sexual orientation and gender expression become standard demographic variables in national random samples.

WHEN DOES MIDLIFE OR OLDER AGE HAPPEN?

The age boundaries for middle adulthood are approximately between forty and sixty-four years of age, with most researchers using age sixty-five as the entry point into older age. The boundaries of these life periods, however, are not clearly definable by age (Bumpass & Aquilino, 1995), stages (Clausen, 1986), or tasks (Rothblum, Mintz, Cowan, & Haller, 1995). Factors that make the boundaries ambiguous are the ever-expanding life expectancy rates and the increasing number of persons working beyond age sixty-five (Herdt, Beeler, & Rawls, 1997).

Most of the gay persons studied by Kerztner (1999) did not experience an abrupt awareness of aging, although many took note of minor changes in physical appearance and stamina. An awareness of being older was signaled for some of the men in this sample by births in extended families or the death of a parent. Many cited an absence of social markers for growing older such as marriage, childbirth, or milestones in the lives of growing children.

HISTORICAL CONTEXTS

Heterosexism

As with all LGBT persons, those who are midlife and older contend with the oppression of stigma and discrimination, including violence ("Homosexuals Said to Face," 1994). Being stigmatized also causes dilemmas in everyday life ranging from holding hands in public to having children to choosing a career (Adelman, 2000).

The concept of heterosexim directly focuses on the experiences of oppression. It was defined by Herek (1995) as "the ideological system that denies, denigrates, and stigmatizes any nonheterosexual form of behavior, identity, relationship, or community" (p. 321). This ideological system operates at both cultural and individual levels. At the cultural level, it is the standard belief that affectional and sexual expression is only acceptable between men and women. This belief is constantly reinforced by social customs and institutions and is so pervasive and accepted that we rarely notice its existence or practices (Herek, 1995).

Another example of cultural heterosexism is how lesbian and gay persons are portrayed in the media. Not until 1969 did LGBT images even appear in film, television, radio, or print media. The stories in early films were primarily of lesbians who were lonely, emotionally unstable, or sex crazed. But in the 1990s, films began to have more positive lesbian and gay characters, and fairly neutral lesbian and gay characters have continued to appear on television. These film and television characters, and celebrity lesbians such as k.d. lang and Melissa Etheridge, are distant, positive models but are better than no positive models. Not all portrayals of LGBT persons are positive; jokes on television game shows continue to include denigrating words when referring to gay persons, such as fruit, queen, and fairy (Jensen, 1999).

Because heterosexism is pervasive in mainstream culture, it is not surprising to see it also operate at the individual level in behaviors and feelings directed at LGBT persons (Herek, 1995). This manifestation can range from jokes and derogatory words to physical attacks and murders (McDougall, 1993; Neisen, 1990). The accompanying feelings include disgust and indignation (e.g., Berrill, 1990; Herek, 1993).

Two core factors that contribute to heterosexism at the individual level are prejudice and stereotypes. Prejudice is a prejudgment or negative bias directed to an entire group of persons although one has limited or no experience with any person in the group (DiAngelo, 1997; Johansson, 1990). Prejudice is maintained by stereotypes (Herek, 1995) that overemphasize specific characteristics of a target group (Yarhouse, 1999). Some stereotypes encompass all subordinated groups such as their inferiority or threat to members of the dominant group. Other stereotypes are specific to a certain group, such as the belief that lesbian and gay persons can influence the sexual orientation of heterosexual persons (Herek, 1995).

Violence

The most extreme reflection of cultural and individual hetero-sexism is violence (e.g. Berrill, 1990; Comstock, 1991; Herek, 1990, 1993). Lesbian and gay persons are a frequent target of bias violence (Dean, Wu, & Martin, 1992; Von Schulthess, 1992). Reviewing twenty-four local, regional, and national samples of LGB persons, Berrill (1992) reported the proportion of different types of harass-ment and violence: assault with weapons (9 percent), physical assault (17 percent), vandalization of property (19 percent), threats of vio-lence (44 percent), objects thrown (25 percent), spit at (13 percent), and verbal harassment (80 percent). One estimate shows that more than 80 percent of transgender persons experience physical assaults because of their sex-gender expression (GenderPAC, 1998).

Though not a significant difference, older LGBT persons report less victimization compared to younger LGBT persons (D'Augelli & Grossman, 2001). They report less verbal abuse, fewer threats of vio-lence, and fewer objects thrown at them during their lifetimes. Yet these persons are victimized. D'Augelli and Grossman (2001) and Grossman, D'Augelli, and O'Connell (2001) studied a national and geographically diverse sample of 416 LGB persons sixty years of age or older (age range: 60-91, median age: 68.5). Most identified as les-bian or gay (92 percent), 8 percent as bisexual. Most were white, 3 percent African American, 2 percent Latino. A third (34 percent) of this group were living in a major urban area, another third (36 per-cent) in a small city, and smaller numbers in a suburb (10 percent), a small town or rural area (13 percent), or other type of community (7 percent). Many of these older pesons had been victimized during their lives. Two-thirds (63 percent) were verbally abused, more than one-quarter (29 percent) was threatened with violence; 16 percent were punched, kicked, or beaten; 11 percent had objects thrown at them; 12 percent were assaulted with a weapon; and 29 percent were threatened with disclosure of their sexual orientation. Twenty percent also reported employment discrimination based on their sexual orientation, and 7 percent reported housing discrimination. Older gay and bisexual men are more likely to report victimization than older lesbian and bisexual women. These numbers are consistent with the results of other studies (e.g., Herek, Gillis, & Cogan, 1999; Otis & Skinner, 1996).

The study reported by D'Augelli and Grossman (2001) and Grossman et al. (2001) showed that support network size when one is older is unrelated to victimization. Nor is there a difference between those living with a partner and those living alone. However, as household income increases, levels of reported victimization decreases. It also increases with greater visibility. The earlier self-identified LGB persons made disclosures to others, the more victimization they recalled experiencing. Those who were members of more LGB organizations or attended them regularly reported more victimization. If being out occurred during less supportive times, physical victimization might have also been more brutal.

Attacks directed toward persons because of same-sex gender sexual orientation have a more powerful negative impact than other crimes. Otis and Skinner (1996) demonstrated that depression was associated with being victimized because of one's sexual orientation. In the studies by D'Augelli and Grossman (2001) and Grossman et al. (2001), being physically attacked because of sexual orientation was especially associated with negative outcomes. The current state of mental health was worse for those who were physically attacked; they also experienced less recent positive change in their mental health. Of those who attempted suicide, more had been physically attacked than had been verbally attacked or not attacked at all. Those who had experienced no sexual-orientation victimization or only verbal attacks had higher self-esteem than those reporting victimization. They also had less internalized oppression leading to suicidal thoughts, compared to those who had experienced physical attacks.

Escalating Violence

Violence directed at lesbian and gay persons is escalating. The National Coalition of Anti-Violence Programs (NCAVP, 2000) is a voluntary network composed of twenty-five community-based programs that monitors and responds to anti-LGBT violence nationwide. The coalition reported violent incidents directed at LGBT persons in

1999 for thirteen cities, states, and regions across the United States. Compared to 1998, reports of anti-LGBT incidents of violence declined slightly (3 percent) (2,017 versus 1,965) in 1999, but only in four of the thirteen reporting regions. Incidents of violence increased at a mean rate of 40 percent in nine other regions between 1998 and 1999. The increases ranged from 7 percent in Columbus, Ohio, to 116 percent in Chicago.

In 2002, 1,968 incidents of anti-LGBT harassment or violence were reported to the National Coalition of Anti-Violence Programs (NCAVP, 2000). The FBI began to track hate crimes motivated by sexual orientation in 1992 and has continued to rank antigay violence as the third most frequent bias-motivated crime. In 2002, it reported that 16.7 percent of the total reported hate crimes (7,462) were motivated by bias related to sexual orientation (Partners Against Hate, 2003). In March 2004, the NCAVP reported that hate violence against lesbian, gay, bisexual, and transgender persons rose 24 percent in the six months following the U.S. Supreme Court's decision in the *Lawrence v. Texas* case (June 26, 2003). This decision struck down all remaining sodomy laws in the United States. Instances in violence rose in six of ten regions surveyed from the beginning of June 2003 through the end of December 2003. The increases included 120 percent in Chicago, 133 percent in Colorado, 43 percent in New York, and 14 percent in San Francisco. In addition, there were significant reversals or downward trends in a number of regions (NCAVP, 2004).

Estimates of bias crimes are most likely inaccurate. This is due to many unreported cases, estimated to be as high as 85 percent (Berrill, 1992). Many bias crimes are not reported because of the stigma associated with them (Waldo, Hesson-McInnis, & D'Augelli, 1998), and for fear of being "outed" or losing control of the management of one's identity (Tewksbury, Grossi, Suresh, & Helms, 1999). Harassment at the hands of police or others is also feared (Herek, 1995; Murphy, 1994).

The perpetrators of bias violence are now bolder. Instead of drive-by verbal slurs, they now use bats, ropes, and knives, and their actions are more premeditated (Ilnytzky, 1999). The most brutal bias violence is murder, and the murders are brutal—such as heads being bashed in or being run over with a car. Murders of LGBT persons increased 13 percent between 1998 and 1999, with a large increase in violent incidents perpetrated by groups of ten or more. In 1999, as in 1998, most offenders (87 percent) were male, and two-thirds were under age thirty (National Coalition of Anti-Violence Programs, 2000). Teenagers are the perpetrators of the most vicious attacks (Savin-Williams, 1994).

Older LGBT Cohorts

The study of lesbian and gay persons across later life reflects the impact of social change over the past three decades. For example, on June 26, 2003, the U.S. Supreme Court struck down laws in Texas and twelve other states that criminalized sex between persons of the same sex-gender (Pusey, 2003). However, today's older LGB persons grew up when heterosexism was unchallenged and the culture and social institutions reflected unquestioned pathological and negative views of "homosexuality" (Grossman et al., 2001). The "gay liberation" movement of the late 1960s and 1970s had not yet occured (Herdt et al., 1997). These older LGB persons had no sense of community or culture to provide contacts, support, resources, role models, or language for same sex-gender attractions (Bohan, 1996). LGBT persons were isolated from one another except for a few small, secret friendship networks and a few clubs and bars in large cities (Herdt et al., 1997). Clubs and bars did not advertise their locations, partly to maintain the patrons' anonymity (James & Murphy, 1998), and the patrons used fictitious names (Henry, 1941). Even in friendship groups, members protected one another by not disclosing names or identities (D'Emilio, 1983).

Some LGBT persons embraced the "homosexual" subculture in bars and frequented them. Unfortunately, bars were often raided by local police who harassed the patrons verbally, physically, and sexually; arrested them; and provided their names to newspapers and employers. This led to loss of jobs, residences, children, and, sometimes, visitation rights with one's children. Often, the parents of these persons disowned them (D'Emilio, 1983; D. Martin & Lyon, 1995).

"Homosexuality," or sexual expressions by two consenting adults of the same sex-gender, was illegal in every state (D'Augelli & Garnets, 1995; D'Emilio, 1983). The police arrested gay persons and charged them with nonviolent offenses such as consensual sodomy, sexual perversion, and public indecency. Both lesbian and gay persons were charged with patronizing gay bars, touching another person of the same sex-gender in public, or wearing the clothing of another sex-gender. Some were sent to prison. When released from prison they were forced to register as sex offenders with their local police departments. Sometimes those arrested were committed to mental hospitals (Bérubé, 1990). Acknowledging their sexual identities to a family physician or psychiatrist could also lead to institutionalization for chronic mental illness (Claes & Moore, 2000).

Older LGBT persons have had different oppressive experiences depending on what cohort they are in or the historical period when they grew up. Those now over age eighty-five make up the fastest growing cohort of LGBT persons in the United States today. They were born before 1917 and reached their twenty-first birthday by 1938. Both lesbian and gay persons served in the armed forces during World War II (Kimmel, 2002) where they discovered others like themselves (Bérubé, 1990; D'Emilio, 1983). In many ways, these experiences led to the beginning of the modern LGB community. However, for some LGB persons the experience in the armed forces was not positive, as they were identified as "homosexual" and discharged from the services. The military got rid of identified "homosexuals" with court marshals and dishonorable discharges (Bohan, 1996; D. Martin & Lyon, 1995). This hindered the ability of these persons to fit back into American society and the workforce. In addition, post-service military benefits were often denied (Loughery, 1998).

Lesbian and gay persons in the cohort now over age seventy were born before 1932 and were in their twenties in 1950 when the U.S. Senate authorized an investigation of "homosexuals" and other "perverts" employed in the government. This was accompanied by a report that claimed that these persons were dangerous because they were predatory and capable of changing heterosexuals into "homosexuals." They were viewed as emotionally unstable, making them amenable to blackmail and extortion; thereby, they endangered national security. That same year, the FBI was charged with supplying the Civil Service commission with background information on applicants and employees. Lists were compiled of "homosexuals" who were fired from or denied jobs. The United States Postal Service tracked persons who received gay erotica or joined gay or lesbian pen pal clubs (D'Emilio, 1983; D. Rosenfeld, 1999).

The FBI established liaisons with vice squad officers who conducted surveillance of gay bars and other "homosexual" gathering places. Federal policy toward "homosexuals" found an ally in state and local police because of a long history of harassing "homosexuals" (D. Rosenfeld, 1999).

This over age seventy cohort was in their twenties when President Eisenhower issued executive order #10450 in 1953 directing that "homosexuals" be dismissed from government jobs (Kimmel, 2002). This order listed "sexual perversion" as sufficient and necessary grounds for dismissal from and disbarment from federal jobs (D'Emilio, 1983). It coincided with the anticommunist hearings of Senator Joe McCarthy, which dictated that any persons working for the federal government suspected of being a communist or a "homosexual" were to be removed from their jobs. "Homosexual" persons were included because "homosexuality" was also linked with subversive activity. The numbers of dismissals for being "homosexual" far exceeded those for real or alleged involvement with the Communist party (Claes & Moore, 2000; Loughery, 1998). "Homosexuals," viewed as a menace and as security risks, were not only sought out and fired from the State Department and other federal agencies but from businesses contracting with the federal government. The military also applied the security standards of the Eisenhower administration to their employees for dismissal of "homosexuals" (D'Emilio, 1983). Military bases were periodically purged of "homosexuals." The expulsion rate increased from 1,000 per year in the late 1940s to 2,000 per year in the early 1950s to 3,000 per year in the early 1960s. Often, court-martial proceedings needed for a dishonorable discharge were bypassed and the expulsions were done through administrative channels in which all that was necessary was that these persons were deemed undesirable. No proof of the charges was required as in court-martial proceedings (D'Emilio, 1983). "Homosexuals" also could not work in many state and local governments, as well as in many institutions and businesses in the private sector (Bohan, 1996; D'Emilio, 1983; Esterberg, 1996).

Midlife Cohorts

Using the age boundaries for midlife of forty to sixty-four, midlife today includes lesbian and gay persons born between 1940 and 1964. They are in several cohorts. Those in the oldest cohort were children during World War II and were teenagers in the 1950s. They were born prior to the end of World War II and would have been over age twenty-four at the time of the Stonewall riots in June 1969. They might have been relatively unaware of this cultural paradigm shift because of isolation.

A second midlife cohort was part of the postwar baby boom. The members were children in the 1950s. In their teen years, the civil rights movement and antiwar activism overlapped. During their early adult years, they could locate a homophile organization that could be called from across the country. Their lives were influenced by the modern LGBT movement that evolved after the Stonewall riots. Lesbians were also influenced by the consciousness-raising experiences associated with the early women's movement.

Members of a third midlife cohort are in their early forties now and entered a quite different adult world from the other two cohorts. For example, couples in this cohort might have commitment ceremonies or get legally married, if living in certain locations in the United States such as Massachusetts or if they travel to several locations in Canada. They might have children through previous heterosexual marriages, adoption, surrogates, or alternative insemination. They might attend large parties for LGBT persons in luxury hotels (Cantu, 2003; Mitchell, 2000).

The midlife generation (especially the second and third cohorts) is charting a new path as the first generation of LGBT persons to reach midlife since the 1969 Stonewall rebellion and the advent of the gay liberation movement (Kimmel & Sang, 1995). Through political, professional, and community actions (some members of this cohort were active participants in the social protests associated with Stonewall), this generation shaped a historical time in which they achieved higher visibility and acceptance and some progress in civil rights protections. Each subsequent generation of LGBT persons will live with more visibility, acceptance, and advances (as well as retreats) in civil rights (Gurevitch, 2000).

THE TURNING POINT OF STONEWALL

During the decade of the 1960s, sexual contact between two persons of the same sex-gender was still a criminal offense in most states (M. P. Levine, 1992). Lesbian and gay persons had some success pursuing the end of some of the oppressions they experienced. For example, they took municipalities to court to end harassment and entrapment by police, to stop bar raids and unnecessary search and seizure, and to stop government actions that shut down lesbian and gay businesses. They claimed that these actions violated the constitutional principles of privacy, due process, and rights of free speech and association. They also challenged the obscenity laws that were used to censor gay materials such as magazines, books, and art (Seidman, 2002). The most important event of this decade, however, was Stonewall.

On the night of June 28, 1969, a riot erupted following a routine police raid and attempt by the police to close down the Stonewall Inn in Greenwich Village because liquor was allegedly sold without a license. The patrons at this bar included local gay persons, "drag queens" (men who dressed in women's clothes), and "butch" lesbians (women who displayed masculine-type behavior). Many racial and ethnic minorities were there that night (Duberman, 1993; Gainor, 1999). Patrons were forced into police vans but were released when the police retreated from thrown bottles and cans. The streets were later cleared when police reinforcement arrived. However, for several days and nights following, hundreds of protesters gathered to support the resistance and to battle the police. Fires were started throughout the West Village and graffiti was written on the boarded-up windows (Bohan, 1996; Faderman, 1991; Herdt & Boxer, 1993; Jost, 2000).

Stonewall was not the first act of resistance by lesbian and gay persons, but it was a watershed event that evoked political activism and became the key symbol of the contemporary lesbian and gay movement (E. Stein, 1999) and of "gay pride" (Bohan, 1996). LGBT persons reframed the problem from themselves to society (Jay & Young, 1972).

Lesbian and gay persons now in their midsixties were in their midthirties at the time of Stonewall in 1969, and the oldest-old (eighty-five) were well into midlife (L. M. Woolf, 2002). Living during the pre-Stonewall years, older LGBT persons did not experience concepts such as "gay pride" (Christian & Keefe, 1997), nor were they energized by calls to be "out" after Stonewall (Wahler & Gabbay, 1997). Although some of these persons were much affected by post-Stonewall developments and were even active in promoting them, they had little relevance for many of them (Cohler & Hostetler, 2002). The cohort of LGBT persons now in midlife, however, is the last generation to have lived their adolescence and young adulthood in hiding. They are living their adulthood in an increasingly public community.

Important historical changes occurred in the 1970s that affected both younger and older cohorts of lesbian and gay persons. The protest and liberation movement of this period transformed the lesbian and gay culture from isolation and fragmentation to group consciousness and collective identity (Cruikshank, 1992). The political scene also changed, including the name applied to post-Stonewall politics: liberationism (e.g., Adam, 1995). Liberationists were critical of the assimilationist politics of the early lesbian and gay groups such as the Mattachine Society and the Daughters of Bilitis because they did not challenge heterosexual domination. The assimilationist agenda, the major strategy of the gay movement, focused on equal treatment and equal rights through reform, not revolution. Liberationists drew strategies that fostered hope for revolutionary change in the oppression perpetrated by a heterosexual dictatorship (Seidman, 2002). The strategies came from the civil rights movement, including black militants who provided models for transforming stigma into pride and strength; the New Left and other movements that provided critiques of American society and models of confrontational political action; and the women's liberation movement that provided political analysis of sexism and sex-gender roles (D'Emilio, 1993). This important change in gay politics, representing the radical branch of the gay liberation movement, focused on the heterosexual society and its institutions rather than on the "homosexual" person. It also called for a civil rights movement for LGBT persons (D. Rosenfeld, 1999).

The early 1970s were exciting years for gay liberation. The Gay Liberation Front and other groups, including the Radical Faeries, the Furies, and Radical Lesbians, published newspapers, newsletters, and books on their ideologies and cultures. Members of these groups marched and organized sit-ins. They appeared on television and met with newspaper editors (Seidman, 2002). Among the various liberationist groups, the Gay Liberation Front (GLF) developed out of the radicalism of the New Left and was the most important group at the time (D. Rosenfeld, 1999). The GLF defined "homosexuals" as an oppressed subordinated group and sought revolutionary change for all oppressed subordinated groups (D'Emilio, 1983) through eradication of oppressive social institutions. Another goal was authenticity or openness about one's sexual identity as the way to liberation from isolation and secrecy (D. Rosenfeld, 1999).

The call to disclose garnered mixed responses. Some people did come out of the closet and into the streets, but others saw gay liberation as, if not more of a threat than heterosexual society, at least an equal one (D. Rosenfeld, 1999). The risks were great; the fate of others who had disclosed was known. Public disclosures, therefore, were not epidemic (Lee, 1977). Many also feared the dissolution of the "homosexual" subculture and what it provided, including a sense of purpose, tradition, and place (D. Rosenfeld, 1999).

By the mid-1970s, the gay movement, still inspired by liberationism, challenged state laws that criminalized sodomy by appealing to a constitutional right to privacy and equal treatment. The gay movement also turned its attention and resources toward gaining the same rights and protections any other citizen. Well-financed professional national organizations such as Lambda Legal Defense, the Lesbian and Gay Task Force, and the Human Rights Campaign made the achievement of equal civil rights their focus. In small towns and large cities across the country, organizations dedicated to gay rights ordinances enactment were formed. However, victories in the 1970s were few as only forty communities passed gay rights ordinances (Seidman, 2002).

Liberationists influenced some shift away from the assimilationism of the previous decades, but they were not successful in mobilizing mass support for their vision (Seidman, 2002). After the mid-1970s, liberationist groups were only a marginal presence (Vaid, 1995). Their dissolution mainly resulted from battles over ideology and strategy. Some LGBT persons wanted reform (e.g, the Gay Activist Alliance), while others, influenced by Marxist or radical feminist rhetoric, wanted a revolution. By the mid-1970s, gay librationism no longer existed as an organized political movement (Seidman, 2002). Yet a liberationist political agendum developed after the onslaught of AIDS (acquired immunodeficiency syndrome) in groups such as ACT UP (AIDS Coalition to Unleash Power), Queer Nation, Lesbian Avengers, and Sex Panic (e.g., Vaid, 1995).

Although the liberationist agenda was not successful, the lesbian and gay culture, inspired by Stonewall, became more cohesive (Cruikshank, 1992). The largest LGBT demonstrations before Stonewall included only a few dozen participants. In June 1970, a march in

New York to commemorate Stonewall included about 5,000 participants (D'Emilio, 1993). Only fifty lesbian and gay organizations existed at the time of Stonewall; more than 700 lesbian and gay groups
existed by 1973. Mostly concentrated in New York City and other urban areas, political activist and civil rights organizations, social
clubs, community centers, businesses, social services organizations,
and newspapers and magazines gained popularity. The new visibility
of lesbian and gay persons, however, had a downside with the
increased attacks by conservative political and religious groups
(D'Augelli & Garnets, 1995).

THE HIV/AIDS EPIDEMIC

Although "gay liberation" was synonymous with a politically
aware identity, it also connoted for many a new community-oriented
identity accompanied by personal, social, and sexual freedom
(Bohan, 1996). This all changed in the 1980s, however, when the
medical and social crises of the HIV (human immunodeficiency virus)/AIDS epidemic became the predominant focus in the lives of urban gay persons. Illness, death, loss of friends and partners, and the
fear of one's own diagnosis pervaded life (Paul, Hays, & Coates,
1995).

Governmental and social agencies were indifferent to the HIV/
AIDS crisis. The gay community, therefore, was challenged to develop ways to care for its own (James & Murphy, 1998). Energetic
volunteerism by both lesbian and gay persons attempted to meet community needs and to refocus existing programs on those with HIV/
AIDS (Omoto & Crain, 1995; Paul et al., 1995). The development of
an array of informal social services, such as self-help and support
groups, supplemented formal social services organizations (D'Augelli,
1989c). Yet because of the immense scope of the epidemic, the community was unable to meet all the needs. Therefore, members of the
gay community participated in considerable political organization to
expand funding for more services and research focused on a cure for
HIV/AIDS (Paul et al., 1995). Organizations such as ACT UP formed
in March of 1987 in New York City, used direct action to obtain what
was necessary, (D. Rosenfeld, 1999).

During the 1990s, HIV/AIDS and the need for more resources still
consumed much of the energy in lesbian and gay communities. Now

the focus broadened to include the lack of legal protections in many areas and the need for civil rights at all levels of government and in business, universities, and other institutions (Paul et al., 1995). These issues continue to be at the forefront of lesbian and gay interests. While Congress continued to block federal civil rights legislation that would include sexual orientation, the Civil Service commission and ultimately an executive order by President Clinton ended legal job discrimination in all federal agencies. By 2000 gay rights ordinances in states and cities were well over 300. Gay rights laws were also being passed in small towns and suburban communities in the Northeast and West, the South, Midwest, and Northwest.

Mandates for domestic partnerships started passing in the mid-1990s and are increasing in states, cities, businesses, and institutions of higher education (Seidman, 2002). Same-sex couples living in California, Connecticut, the District of Columbia, Hawaii, Maine, and New Jersey can take advantage of domestic partner laws. (HRC, 2004). The benefits are variable, however, with some plans providing substantive financial benefits while other plans include only bereavement and/or family leave, and other plans only a membership such as at a gym.

Greater benefits for lesbian and gay persons come with civil unions and far more with legal marriage. State legislatures can create civil unions for same sex-gender couples. This is the case in Vermont, which is the only state to offer (starting in mid-2000) same sex-gender couples the state-level rights and benefits given to heterosexual couples. Domestic partnership laws in California and New Jersey provide benefits similar to those provided in civil unions, but both stop short of the full provisions in civil unions. Even full provisions of a civil union are limited, however, as civil unions do not provide the federal-level rights, benefits, and protections that come with a civil marriage license. More than 1,000 federal rights and privileges that married couples receive automatically are withheld from "civil unionized" couples because of the federal Defense of Marriage Act (DOMA) which prohibits the federal government from recognizing civil unions. Nor are civil unions necessarily recognized in states that have no civil union law (Religious Tolerance.org, 2004; Lesbian Life, 2004b).

Many lesbian and gay persons want the right to legally marry in order to get all the rights that come with this arrangement. However, civil unions and particularly the beginning developments allowing same sex-gender marriage go against the urging of the gay liberation movement for lesbian and gay persons to reject heterosexual normative behaviors such as marriage (Whitman, 1992). Yet, given the increasing assimilation of lesbian and gay persons into mainstream culture it seems that a lesbian and gay life course is emerging that closely follows heterosexual norms (Hostetler, 2000). The push for gay marriage, therefore, is in full swing, although there are forceful obstacles.

Until recent years, same sex-gender couples could not marry anywhere in the world. However, in 2001, Holland expanded its definition of marriage to include both opposite-sex and same sex-gender couples. This happened in Belgium in 2003 (although adoption of children is not allowed); in Ontario in 2003; and in British Columbia, Quebec, and the territory of Yukon in Canada in 2004. Movements are underway to allow same sex-gender marriage in Manitoba and Nova Scotia (Religious Tolerance.org, 2004).

The Netherlands has full marriage and registered partnership rights for same sex-gender or opposite-sex couples. France has a civil solidarity pact which grants same sex-gender or opposite-sex partners rights of next-of-kin, inheritance, social security, and tax benefits. Portugal grants partnership rights to same sex-gender and opposite-sex couples. Partnership rights include next-of-kin, inheritance, property, social security, and tax benefits. Denmark has registered partnerships for same sex-gender couples who are granted the same rights as married couples. Germany recognizes next-of-kin and property inheritance rights for same sex-gender couples who register as partners. The newly elected prime minister of Spain has promised to give same-sex unions the same rights and privileges as heterosexual unions (Lesbian Life, 2004a). Gay marriage was approved at an October 1, 2004, cabinet meeting (Reuters, 2004).

In the United States, only a man and a woman can have a marriage recognized by their state except for lesbian and gay residents of Massachusetts who won a court battle for the right to marry. In 2003, the Massachusetts Supreme Judicial Court issued a ruling demanding that the legislature pass a law authorizing same-sex marriages. The first licenses were issued in Cambridge on May 17, 2004 (Lesbian Life, 2004a).

Same-sex couples could obtain marriage licenses in San Francisco and in various towns in New Mexico and New York for short intervals of time during 2004. However, none could register their marriages. Also, the California Supreme Court ordered San Francisco to stop issuing marriage licenses, so same sex-gender marriage is no longer an option there for now. The San Francisco licenses were also nullified by the California Supreme Court, which ruled they had been issued without legal authority (Kravets, 2004).

Multnomah County, Oregon, which includes Portland, began issuing same-sex marriage licenses in 2004. However, a judge ordered the county to stop issuing the licenses to gay and lesbian couples until the state legislature rules on the matter. All the marriages that were performed between March 3 and April 20, however, were considered legal. Same sex-gender marriages were held in New Paltz, New York, in 2004 but were suspended soon after this began. New Jersey married its first gay couple on March 8, 2004, but on March 9 the state's attorney general ordered officials to stop performing same sex-gender marriages or face criminal charges. He also declared the licenses issued invalid. Although lesbian and gay persons cannot get married in Seattle or San Jose, California, these cities recognize same-sex marriages performed in other places, including Canada, San Francisco, or Portland, Oregon (Lesbian Life, 2004a).

Since the Massachusetts ruling, more than thirty-seven states have introduced legislation aimed at preserving the traditional definition of marriage as a union between a man and a woman. Only five states have no laws that prohibit same sex-gender marriage (Religious Tolerance.org, 2004). Those who oppose gay marriage are also trying to get constitutional amendments passed in their states blocking same sex-gender marriages by short-circuiting court decisions. In a statewide vote August 3, 2004, Missouri adopted a constitutional ban against gay marriage as did Louisiana on September 18, 2004. This had already happened in Alaska, Hawaii, Nebraska, and Nevada. Similar amendments likely will be on the ballots in many other states (Stateline.org, 2004).

President George W. Bush is trying to get an amendment passed to ban gay marriage. So, although many lesbian and gay persons want to be legally married, the right to do this is in a highly fluid state. As noted, some couples have been married only to have their marriages voided.

Although legal reforms are advancements, they have not made LGBT persons equal citizens. In addition, most cities and states lack laws that protect these persons from housing and job discrimination. As yet, the Employment Non-Discrimination Act (ENDA), first introduced in Congress in 1994, has not passed. Jobs and homes of most LGBT persons are not legally protected by any local, state, or federal laws. Moreover, antigay legislation exists in hundreds of cities. Government policies such as "Don't ask, don't tell" in the armed forces and the Defense of Marriage Act underscore the second-class citizenship status of lesbian and gay persons (Seidman, 2002).

PART I:
FINDING OUT WHO ONE IS
AND TELLING OTHERS

Chapter 1

Concepts, Identities, and Terms

GENDER AND SEX

Although terminology is discussed in the last section of this chapter and in subsequent chapters, the terms *gender* and *sex (sex-gender)* require clarification at this point because they appear throughout the book. These terms seem to be the same but they are not; what each term supposedly represents is questionable. The standard use of the term *sex* distinguishes males and females by mostly biological characteristics (Rutter & Schwartz, 2000). Genitalia, chromosomes, reproductive organs, gametes, hormones, and other biological characteristics assign a person to the category of male or female, although this determination is usually made on genital appearance alone (Devor, 2002). Biological factors used to classify persons as male or female do not divide persons into two distinct groups (Coombs, 1998). This is evident in intersex persons who are born with different combinations of genitals, chromosomes, and secondary sex characteristics (e.g., body hair, breasts). These combinations are not clearly classifiable as male or female (E. Stein, 1999). So, there is confusion: Is it a boy or a girl? (Chase, 2002; Lombardi, 2001). This situation happens in about 1 in 2,000 births (Feinberg, 1996).The social as well as legal sex status of intersex persons may be determined by legal opinion, medical practitioners, or government bureaucrats (Devor, 2002). The sex assignment for others may also be questionable such as an XY (chromosomal) baby who has external female genitals but will never fully develop internal female sexual organs (Maurer, 1999). Adding to the complexity, some cultures recognize more than two sexes (e.g., Blackwood, 1984). The standard use of the term *gender* (feminine or masculine) determines social status based on what society expects or because of one's assigned sex (Maurer, 1999). However, gender can be imposed on experiences that may have no relation to the sex of a person (Bohan & Russell, 1999b; McKenna & Kessler, 2000).

In this text, the term *sex-gender* is adapted from E. Stein (1999) to indicate the complex and unsettled issues surrounding sex and gender. Sex-gender includes all the characteristics (for example, biological, psychological, cultural) that distinguish males-men from females-women, although current views about what biological features distinguish males from females may be inaccurate.

SEXUAL ORIENTATION

Two important issues about sexual orientation are how to define it and the practice of dividing it along binary lines. Although there are multiple definitions of sexual orientation, E. Stein (1999) proposed that the disposition definition is the most suitable one because it incorporates the virtues of two other definitions: (1) behavior and (2) self-identification. Accordingly, sexual orientation first represents one's sexual behaviors as well as sexual desires and sexual fantasies. For example, a person may have desires and fantasies about having sex primarily with others of the same sex-gender. This person is likely to engage in sexual acts primarily with others of the same sex-gender, but not always. Adding the second part of the definition, self-identification, means that one also adopts a sexual identity such as gay or lesbian. As discussed later, one's sexual identity and sexual orientation are usually in sync, but not always.

Another issue regarding sexual orientation is that researchers and others typically dichotomize persons by sexual attractions (same sex-gender or other sex-gender), sex-gender identity (male or female), and sex-gender role (masculine or feminine) (Firestein, 1996). As suggested already, however, binary divisions such as these may not be accurate (E. Stein, 1999). They may not reflect sexual behaviors or be stable over time. Alfred A. Kinsey and his associates (Kinsey, Pomeroy, & Martin, 1948; Kinsey, Pomeroy, Martin, & Gebbard, 1953) discovered that persons often display more of a mix of "homosexual" and heterosexual sexual behaviors rather than one or the other. This prompted the Kinsey group to develop a seven-point bipolar continuum to rate sexual orientation. Positioning on this continuum depends upon the proportion a person's sexual behavior is oriented to one or the other sex-gender. This proportion is placed on a range from 0 (exclusive heterosexual behavior) to a midpoint of 3 (equal heterosexual and "homosexual" behaviors) to 6 (exclusive "homosexual" behavior). These scores, however, are not stable, as they can vary at different times in one's life (Kinsey et al., 1948).

Sexual behavior theory was revolutionized by the Kinsey scale that undermined traditional restrictive views (V. L. Bullough, 1994b; Dynes & Donaldson, 1992). A startling finding of the Kinsey studies was a greater incidence of same sex-gender sexual behavior than was formerly believed to exist. Substantial numbers of persons participated in both same sex-gender and other sex-gender sexual activity. About 50 percent of men and 28 percent of women reported some degree of same sex-gender sexual experience in their lives, although after adolescence only 4 to 5 percent of men and less than 3 percent of women reported exclusively same sex-gender sexual activity. Based on cross-cultural studies done about the same time, Ford (1948) and Ford & Beach (1951) found that some degree of same sex-gender sexual behavior was "normal" in seventy-six human societies.

Although the Kinsey studies were revolutionary (V. L. Bullough, 1994b), they were also controversial because of notable shortcomings in theory, methodology, reported findings, and interpretations of findings (V. L. Bullough, 1998; Laumann, Gagnon, Michael, & Michaels, 1994; Sell, 1996). The seven-point scale essentially continued to divide persons into heterosexual or "homosexual" categories. This makes the scale problematic for those who report that they could potentially become sexually involved with both women and men or that they experienced former sexual relationships with both women and men (E. Stein, 1999). Although the middle of the scale was a default category for bisexual experiences, it was ignored (Guidry, 1999; E. Stein, 1999). Yet compared to same sex-gender attractions or sexual behaviors, more men and women display bisexual attractions and sexual behaviors (Kinsey et al., 1948; Kinsey et al., 1953; Laumann et al., 1994; Rogers & Turner, 1991).

Persons who claim a bisexual identity confront a number of myths about their identity, such as "there is no such thing," "bisexual attractions are temporary," or persons who claim that they are bisexual are just experimenting or acting trendy (Guidry, 1999; Rust, 1996a; Udis-Kessler, 1996). These persons often seem indecisive for refusing to admit their real sexual orientation (heterosexual, lesbian, or gay) (Firestein, 1996; R. L. Pope & Reynolds, 1991). As a result of these kinds of distortions, many bisexual persons may repress their bisexual behaviors, feelings, and fantasies or may feel forced to choose an identity that is not bisexual (Paul, 1992; Rust, 1996a; Zook, 2001).

Modifications to Kinsey's work started in the 1970s including, for example, additional factors; measurement of the intensity level of emotional and sexual attractions; and development of two continuous scales with separate ratings, one for measurement of same sex-gender attractions and behaviors, the other for measurement of other sex-gender attractions and behaviors (e.g., Coleman, 1987; Klein, Sepekoff, & Wolf, 1985; Sell, 1996; Shively & De Cecco, 1977; Storms, 1980). None of the scale developments so far have incorporated a multidimensional view of sexual identity. In addition, a thorough factor analysis has not been done. Nor do any of the scales accommodate multiple sex-genders. For example, do transgender or intersex persons constitute a second sex-gender or a third or a fourth? If so, where do we locate them on scales? Where do we locate men and women who experience attraction to intersex or transgender persons (E. Stein, 1999)? Where do we locate transgender persons who experience attractions to men, women, or other transgender persons, and who may sexually interact with gay, lesbian, bisexual, and heterosexually identified others? (Bockting, 1999). Although we know more about sexual orientation now, many questions remain unanswered. The range of sexual interests under the heading of sexual orientation may be too narrow (E. Stein, 1999).

SEXUAL IDENTITY

Whereas sexual orientation has to do with sexual dispositions, sexual desires, and sexual behaviors, sexual identity (e.g., "I am gay" or "I am heterosexual") comes from a given cultural and historical pool of potential sexual identities (Ellis & Mitchell, 2000). We typically expect that the identity one selects is concordant with one's sexual disposition, sexual desire, and sexual behavior. Yet we cannot draw this conclusion with any certainty because various factors are used by persons to determine sexual identity.

Using factors such as sexual desire, sexual behavior (E. Stein, 1999), affectional desire (Shively, Jones, & De Cecco, 1983-1984), and community participation (Golden, 1987), we can see that nothing is definite in predicting identity from these components, either singly or in various combinations. They are independent of one another (Hunter & Hickerson, 2003). For example, some persons claim same sex-gender sexual desire but do not claim a lesbian, gay, or bisexual identity and vice versa. Some persons may be attracted to others of the same sex-gender but never act on the attraction or identify as lesbian, gay, or bisexual. Sometimes women have "romantic friendships" or are psychologically or emotionally passionate about other women but not sexually involved with them (e.g., Faderman, 1981; Rothblum & Brehony, 1993; Rupp, 1997) and do not identify as lesbian. Some women experience affectional desire for a same sex-gender partner and identify themselves as lesbian but may not want sex with this partner (Esterberg, 1997; Peplau & Cochran, 1990). Community participation is sometimes incongruent with sexual behavior and sexual identity.

Each person experiences a unique combination of erotic and affectional desires, emotional attachments, behaviors, fantasies, relationships, and community ties (Rothblum, 2000). There can probably never be enough categories to represent the diversity among people (Horowitz & Newcomb, 2001). M. Diamond (2003) found in a group of eighty nonheterosexual young women (ages eighteen to twenty-five) studied over five years that some experienced difficulty in fitting their personal experiences into rigid sexual identity categories. Diverse experiences cannot easily be lumped together into a few categories. Many women change their sexual identities because they do not feel comfortable with the rigid "boxes" of lesbian or bisexual. As indicated by Russell and Bohan (1999), a set of discrete categories of sexual identities is meaningless.

Variations of sexual identity often occur in ethnic/racial cultures. Persons in different cultures may experience sexual attractions and involvements with persons of the same sex-gender but may not identify as gay, lesbian, or bisexual. No sexual identities in East Asian cultures are analogous to the modern Western constructs of lesbian and gay identities (Chan, 1997). It is especially common for men in Latino cultures who engage in sex with same sex-gender persons to not label themselves as gay or "homosexual," especially if they take the masculine active sexual role of inserter (Carballo-Digéuez, 1989; Espin, 1984). This situation also occurs in some Native American communities. If a male is masculine, the sex-gender of a sexual partner is irrelevant. But, a male who takes the role of a passive, receptive partner while experiencing sex with another male gets tagged with a "homosexual" label (Tofoya, 1996). Bisexual sexual practices are also acceptable in Latino cultures although for some Latino men, these practices hide a same sex-gender sexual orientation (Manalansan, 1996).

Some persons feel that their internal sex-gender identity and their sexual anatomy do not match. For example, a person in a male body may believe that his sex-gender identity is female (Maurer, 1999). Often, persons who feel that their sex-gender identity does not match their biological sex cross-dressed throughout childhood and adolescence. Later they attempt to pass as a member of the sex-gender they wish to be (Seil, 1996). From a sample of men who wished for their sexual anatomy to match their sex-gender, Gagné, Tewksbury, and McGaughey (1997) found that most (thirteen) of the respondents began to cross-dress in childhood, but a few (four) began this activity in adolescence. These men wore women's clothing to relax and to express their "feminine" selves. The motivation for cross-dressing for many of these men was erotic, but this desire dissipated over time for some cross-dressers. Far more important was trying to overcome the discrepancy they felt between their sex-gender and sexual anatomy (Green, 1987; Zuger, 1984).

Adults who wish for their sexual anatomy to match their sex-gender report that they always had, as early as age three to about age ten, strong feelings that they belonged to the other sex-gender (e.g., Gagné et al., 1997; Seil, 1996). If they are willing to go through sex-reassignment surgery (SRS) to change their sex-gender and can finance it, they can experience a match in their sexual anatomy and sex-gender (J. M. Bailey, 1996). Although SRS cannot change a person's chromosomal sex, it can remove internal genital structures, alter external genitalia, and, combined with hormone treatments, dramatically affect a person's secondary sex characteristics. Intersex persons who have ambiguous genitals at birth often undergo surgical reconstruction, usually in infancy. Later in life, however, they may discover the surgically assigned sex-gender does not match their internally desired sex-gender identity (Mauer, 1999; E. Stein, 1999). Many trangender persons conform well to the gender expectations of their sex-gender after SRS and can pass as that sex-gender unnoticed. Other transgender persons, however, cannot pass easily because of their lack of sex-gender conformity or inability to meet the expectations of others about how their sex-gender is expressed (Devor, 2002).

Currently, SRS is not an inevitable step for persons who experience discrepancies between sexual anatomy and internal sex-gender. They may not seek major biological changes but instead lesser changes such as breast implants and electrolysis (B. Bullough & V. Bullough, 1997; Coombs, 1998; Tewksbury & Gagné, 1996). More persons realize that they can live as transgender persons or pass as the other sex-gender without extensive changes in sexual anatomy (Bockting, 1999; Denny, 1997; Gagné & Tewksbury, 1999). SRS is not a requirement but an option (Denny, 2002).

UNSETTLED TERMINOLOGY

Terminology for LGBTI persons varies across geographical areas, cultures, time periods (American Psychological Association [APA], 1991; Donovan, 1992), and from inside and outside LGBTI populations. For example, "homosexual" was by far the most predominant term applied to persons with same sex-gender attractions for more than a century (Herdt & Boxer, 1992). In the past few decades, it has been dropped by most lesbian and gay persons because of its association with negative stereotypes and its use as a pathological diagnosis. It has been replaced with community terms.

Community Terms

Until gay liberation in the late 1960s, "homosexuals" had limited vocabulary through which to understand themselves. They saw their sexual desires as a condition to be suppressed and many got into heterosexual marriages as a way to hide their condition. Others engaged in sexual, social, and emotional relations with other gay or lesbian persons but still understood that their "homosexuality" was a pathological or immoral condition (D. Rosenfeld, 1999). However, profound changes in the meaning of same sex-gender desire or sex-gender expressions occurred and were accompanied by various terminological shifts (Hostetler & Herdt, 1998).

Gay

Following the 1969 Stonewall rebellion, lesbian and gay persons replaced the term *homosexual* with the alternate term *gay*. This term was chosen because of the "refusal to be named by, judged by, or controlled by the dominant majority" (Cruikshank, 1992, p. 91). By the 1980s *gay* was the standard community term (Herdt and Boxer, 1992), but now it applies primarily to males; in this book *gay* designates males.

Lesbian

There is no historical record regarding the origins of the terms *gay* or *lesbian*. The most likely source for *lesbian* was the home of the Greek poet Sappho who lived on the island of Lesbos around 600 B.C. (Money, 1998; Nakayama & Corey, 1993). By the 1980s women wanted a name of their own because of the primary association of the term gay with men (Cruikshank, 1992). *Lesbian* was the chosen term. Women wanted this name to represent their distinct and separate experiences, culture, and community (Jeffreys, 1994; Kennedy & Davis, 1993; T. S. Stein, 1993). By the late 1980s, groups for both women and men usually included *lesbian* in the group name (Cruikshank, 1992).

Bisexual

Bisexual was not a term chosen by the community, but it is acceptable to bisexual persons. The term is used in current affirmative books, networks, and other resources on bisexual persons, as is the shorter version, *bi*. *Bisexualities* is sometimes used to represent the wide diversity among bisexual persons (Stokes & Damon, 1995).

Intersex

As noted earlier, some persons are born with ambiguity in sexual differentiation. *Intersex* is the term applied to persons in this situation. It is a clinical term that emerged in the nineteenth century and has largely replaced the older clinical term *hermaphrodite* (Feinberg, 1996).

Transgender

Clinical terms were also imposed on transgender persons by medical outsiders that implied pathology such as *transvestite, transsexual,* or *sexual dysphoria* (Denny, 1999). The term *transgender* came into widespread use in the 1990s. It now applies to almost anyone who resists gender stereotypes or transgresses sex-gender norms through sexual orientation (gay, lesbian, and bisexual persons) or sex-gender (women who are not stereotypical "feminine" or men who are not stereotypical "masculine") (Denny, 1999; Devor, 2002). The term also includes intersex persons (Carroll & Gilroy, 2002).

Racial and Ethnic LGBT Persons and Terminology

Most research on LGBT persons in racial and ethnic groups includes those who are African American, Asian American, Latino, and Native American. In this book, the terms generally used for these groups are those recommended by the *APA Publication Manual* (2001): black or African American, Latino, Asian American, and Native or Native American. Racial and ethnic persons may prefer other terms such as Chicana/Chicano, Mexican American, or person of color (Martinez, 1998).

Ethnic and racial groups may or may not use the same terms used in the white lesbian and gay communities. Some African-American women, for example, reject the term *lesbian* because it is Eurocentric (Mason-John & Khambatta, 1993). Many Native American persons identify with the terms lesbian, gay, bisexual, transgender, or queer (Tofoya, 1996), but others in this group find these categories too confining. They may prefer one of several "sex-gender styles" that exist among Native Americans such as *not-men* (biological women who perform some male roles) or *not-women* (biological men who perform some female roles) (L. B. Brown, 1997). The term *two spirit* is also used among some Native Americans because it represents more of a spiritual-social identity or an integration of alternative sexuality, alternative sex-gender, and Native American spirituality (Tofoya, 1996, 1997).

Emerging Terms

The term *queer* recently reemerged as a preferred label within some LGBT communities. But this is a controversial term because of politically radical associations (e.g., "Queer Nation"), past uses by heterosexuals to taunt LGB persons (Jeffreys, 1994), and particularly derogatory definitions (e.g., unusual, abnormal, worthless, or counterfeit) (Bryant & Demian, 1998). Queer is also a generic word and, as argued by Jeffreys (1994), generic words typically only refer to men. On the other hand, Khayatt (2002) makes the point that queer was reclaimed to cover all those marginalized because they transgress the norm of sex-genders or sexualities. Yet it is not entirely acceptable or comprehensive enough to cover all the differences it presumes to name. Because the term has no boundaries it may be too loose.

Other changing identifications include *bisensual* (indicating a sensuality that expresses human connecting more accurately than genital sex does), *polysexual* or *polyamorous* (indicating separation of sexuality from sex-gender and sexual dichotomies), and *polyfidelitous* (indicating fidelity to a group of three or more persons) (Rust, 1996a).

The transgender movement also is defining itself beyond the existing terminology (Maurer, 1999). Words or terms created to describe the experiences of these persons including *two spirit* (from Native American traditions), *gender blender, gender bender, gender outlaw, androgyne, drag king,* and *drag queen* (Bockting, 1999; Cole, Denny, Eyler, & Samons, 2000; Maurer, 1999). *Bigender* is a term applied to persons who identify as both man and woman. *Radical transgender, ambigenderist,* and *third sex* are terms applied to sex radicals or those who challenge not just their own sex-gender but the existing sex-gender system (Gagné et al., 1997).

Other combined terms include *lesbian-identified bisexual* and *bisexual lesbian.* They imply a previous lesbian identification or a political commitment to women or to the lesbian community may have existed (Rust, 1995), or there might have been sexual involvement with women and identification as lesbians, but also sexual desire for men. Some women once identified as lesbian and were sexually involved with women, but this is not the case now so they consider themselves to be *transient lesbians.* Sexually, they are now involved with men (Golden, 1996).

We must be sensitive to what persons want to be called and aware that this can change over time. Language sensitivity also applies to intersex persons who may or may not accept the label of intersex.

No terms should be used that perpetuate old stereotypes (Bernstein, 1992). The Committee on Lesbian and Gay Concerns of the APA identified acceptable terminology in 1991, and some of these terms are now in the *APA Publication Manual* (2001). *Homo-*

sexual(s) or *homosexuality* are terms that perpetuate old stereotypes. They appear here in the context of historical discussions and past research, but they are in quotation marks to indicate that they are not acceptable terms. The exception would be if anyone preferred to be called "homosexual." Examples of other unacceptable terms include *preoperative, postoperative,* and *nonoperative* because they imply that SRS overshadows everything else in a transgender person's life. *Transsexual* is also no longer an acceptable term (Denny, 1997).

It might be better if terms such as these were used as adjectives rather than nouns and applied to behaviors rather than to persons. The term *gay,* for example, might apply to someone who experiences regular sexual partners of the same sex-gender but not to someone who's sexual experiences are mainly heterosexual but who on occasion has sex with someone of the same sex-gender (M. Diamond, 2002).

OTHER TERMS

Other terms used in this book also require discussion. The terms *coming out* and *disclosure* are often used interchangeably, but they are separate processes. In this book coming out refers to the internal process of same sex-gender identity development, whereas disclosure refers to the revelation of one's identity to others (Strommen, 1989). A concept recommended by Longres (2000), *subordinated group(s),* is used instead of *minority group(s).* The terms *problem* and *problems* are often presented in quotes or replaced with the terms *difficulty* or *difficulties.* Problem-oriented terminology is less acceptable now because of the emphasis on the strengths of persons. The terms *therapy* and *therapist(s)* are usually in quotes because they signify a narrow approach to what clients may require. The terms *practice* and *practitioner(s)* are more often used. Additional alternative terminology is discussed in several other chapters.

SUMMARY

Sexual orientation is an elusive concept. Currently, the dispositional view of sexual orientation is useful as it includes a person's desires, fantasies, and behaviors. Although there are multivariate scales to measure sexual orientation, none is fully acceptable to date. Gender and sex are also elusive concepts, and the use of sex-gender indicates that issues regarding these concepts are not settled. Sexual identity involves labeling oneself such as lesbian or heterosexual. This labeling process is highly influenced by one's social location and culture. Labels or terms are also variable and change over time. To avoid errors, it is best to ask individuals what terms they apply to themselves.

Chapter 2

Coming Out and Disclosure

STAGES OF THE COMING-OUT PROCESS

Coming out is the experience of separation or differentiation from a heterosexual sexual orientation (Burch, 1997). This is an internal process until one discloses his or her nonheterosexual identity to others. Alternative terms for this process include *identity development* and *sexual questioning* (Savin-Williams & Diamond, 1999).

Decades of research on the coming-out process indicate that most persons come out during the teenage years and early twenties (for example, Chapman & Brannock, 1987; Harry, 1993; Rosario et al., 1996). This timing is especially prevalent among urban, collegiate, and media-saturated communities (e.g., D'Augelli & Hershberger, 1993; Savin-Williams, 1998a). Others may not come out until midlife or later.

Various models have been developed to describe what happens in the coming-out process. Only a few of these models, however, have been subjected to empirical investigation, including the Sexual Identity Formation Model developed by Cass (1979, 1984, 1996), and the Dual-Branch model (Fassinger & Miller, 1996; McCarn & Fassinger, 1996). These models present a linear sequence of three to seven stages (Cohen & Savin-Williams, 1996). Jensen (1999) identified four of the most common stages:

1. Increasing acceptance of a gay or lesbian label as applying to oneself
2. Increasing change in feelings from negative to positive about this self-identity
3. Increasing desire to inform gay, lesbian, and heterosexual persons of one's self-identity
4. Increasing involvement with the lesbian and gay community

Based on longitudinal data from a sample of bisexual men and women in San Francisco, four broad stages of bisexual identity development have been proposed:

1. Initial confusion or inability to make sense of one's bisexuality, uncertain about which sexual category one fits in, experiencing isolation
2. Finding and applying the label to oneself, lessening confusion, positive sexual experiences with both men and women, acceptance of attraction to both sex-genders, finding support from others
3. Settling into the identity or a more complete self-labeling, greater self-acceptance, continued support from others resulting in a more consolidated sense of bisexual self-identification
4. Continued uncertainty about one's sexual identity (M. S. Weinberg, Williams, & Prior, 1994, 1998).

Even if transgender persons do not come out as lesbian, gay, or bisexual, they will experience coming out as transgender and might disclose this identity to others. In a volunteer sample of sixty-five male-to-female (MF) persons, the transition of coming out or "crossing over" from one sex-gender category to another included several tasks:

1. Dealing with the struggles that result from society's negative reaction to what feels natural
2. Discovering names for one's feelings
3. Finding others who are experiencing similar feelings, the most common factor leading to acceptance of identity (Gagné et al., 1997; Gagné & Tewksbury, 1999)

All coming-out models have limitations. Most evolved from clinical and anecdotal data and the stages were usually conceptualized after data collection (Gruskin, 1999). Research samples were small or unrepresentative, and the measures unsound or undeveloped (Fassinger, 1994). Early models may not generalize beyond the cohorts that entered adolescence in the 1960s and 1970s (Herdt, 1992). In addition, some persons do not go through the predicted order of stages or go through every stage. They may skip stages, repeat stages, or get stuck in a stage indefinitely. They can also abort the process altogether and retain a heterosexual identity (e.g., Rust, 1993; Savin-Williams & Diamond, 1999). Some persons have no memory of any coming-out process and instead experience a sudden awareness of their sexual orientation, becoming comfortable with it quickly (Savin-Williams, 1998a).

Although linear coming-out models with stages suggest that once one reaches the end stage identity development ends, for most persons this development is a lifelong process. Some of the models also propose that activism and a politicized public identity signify developmental maturity (Esterberg, 1997; Rust, 1996a). These prescriptions, however, do not recognize the social realities of diverse groups or contexts that may present obstacles for these developments (e.g., work settings, family situations, racial and ethnic backgrounds, geographical locations) or other realities including legal and economic situations and the availability of support systems (Fassinger, 1991; Fassinger & Miller, 1996). Another limitation of coming-out models is the lack of pieces, including social class, race and ethnicity, acculturation or immigration status, bisexual orientation, transgender identity, adolescence, older persons, or categories other than the cognitive category of identity development.

Most of the models are essentialist, indicating that one's sexual orientation is intrinsic to oneself and awaits to come forth. In a sample of older LGB adults studied by Cohler and Hostetler (2002), many presumed that sexual orientation was a fixed and essential characteristic. They believed they had always been lesbian or gay. Rarely are coming-out models based on the constructionist perspective which views sexual identity as a social construction or an interpretation of personal and sociopolitical experiences (Russell & Bohan, 1999) or historical, cultural, or interactional contexts (D. Rosenfeld, 2003). For example, the lesbian and gay rights movement, a new romantic or sexual relationship, or meeting a bisexual person may cause reconstruction of one's experiences through a lesbian, gay, or bisexual filter (Rust, 1996a). Historical location can also influence in opening up or suppressing one's awareness of and access to others like oneself. For example, from interviews with lesbians born between 1917 and 1972, Parks (1999) discovered that across three generations internal progression from self-awareness to self-identification as lesbian was linked to each respondent's awareness of and access to other lesbians and lesbian-identified events. The three generations included the pre-Stonewall era, age forty-five and older; the gay liberation era, ages thirty to forty-four; and the gay rights era, age thirty and younger. Isolation and silence were experienced by lesbians in the pre-Stonewall era and condemnation in the gay liberation era. These experiences were not as prevalent during the gay rights era, and women were more open to identifying as lesbian and had more access to other lesbians. The constructionist perspective does not reject the essentialist perspective but rather points to other influential experiences such as those mentioned that can impact the coming-out process (Russell & Bohan, 1999).

Another missing piece in most coming-out models is the limited focus on females. Models developed for gay persons or the male-oriented "master narrative" of identity development do not fit lesbian and bisexual females (L. M. Diamond, 1996; Savin-Williams, 1998a). Instead, females are more likely to be influenced by current circumstances and choices instead of by early-life predictors as are gay men. The identity process for lesbians is more fluid and ambiguous compared to the more abrupt process reported by gay men (e.g., Gonsiorek, 1993, 1995; T. S. Stein, 1993). Females (both lesbian and bisexual) tend to become aware of their same-gender attractions while in an affectionate relationship with another female, but before sexual involvement (L. M. Diamond, 1998; Esterberg, 1994; M. S. Weinberg et al., 1994). For males, this awareness usually happens following sexual experiences and not necessarily in the context of a close relationship (Dubé, 1997; Nichols, 1990). Females may also delay identifying as lesbian or bisexual because expressions of affection between females are not unusual behaviors. They may need other kinds of interpersonal situations to reinterpret their feelings and take on a lesbian or bisexual identity (Savin-Williams & Diamond, 2000). Once they experience same sex-gender attractions they are less threatened by them than are males (de Monteflores & Schultz, 1978; Marmor, 1980). Although many older white gay persons followed the male-oriented "master narrative," younger cohorts of white gay and bisexual men are less likely to follow it (Dubé, 1997). There may be a master or dominant narrative for particular cohorts (Plummer, 1995), but there may also be significant intracohort variation as well (Cohler & Hostetler, 2002).

COMING OUT IN MIDLIFE AND LATER

Many LGB persons who came out later in life were heterosexually married (e.g., Bell & Weinberg, 1978; Gundlach & Riess, 1968; Saghir & Robbins, 1973; Sang, 1991). In Bradford and Ryan's (1991) survey sample of midlife lesbians, 34 percent were heterosexually married in the past and 4 percent were still married. One-third of divorced men and more than three-fourths of divorced lesbians studied by Bozett (1993) were unaware of their same sex-gender attractions at the time of their marriages.

When same sex-gender desires are first felt when younger, some women decide to return to or not venture from pursuing a heterosexual partnership because of the costs of social stigma and/or the potential loss of motherhood (Kirkpatrick, 1989b). Ponse (1980) discovered some married women with no same sex-gender sexual experience but who identified as lesbian because of fantasies about other women. They also, however, suppressed both the desires and identification. When desires for other women are suppressed, they may return during a reevaluation process in midlife; this time women choose to pursue them (Kirkpatrick, 1989b). For other women the pull toward same sex-gender attraction is so strong that they must pursue these relationships despite the adverse social pressures (Faderman, 1991).

Several studies addressed once-married lesbians in some detail. Twenty-four women who came out later in life were interviewed by Jensen (1999). They primarily lived in the Twin Cities of Minneapolis and St. Paul, Minnesota, and ranged in age from twenty-nine to fifty-eight. Most of these women were married for many years before they made a change in self-identification. Fifteen did not know of their same sex-gender feelings before they married. The other nine described serious attractions to women after they were married but before they came out as lesbians. Seven had varying degrees of awareness, from a fleeting thought to full same sex-gender experiences. For some of the women, attractions occurred before they realized what they meant. The attractions were not necessarily sexual or recognized this way. Four of the women consciously repressed attractions because they thought they were unacceptable or did not know how to interpret them. Some tried to hide their attractions, primarily because they believed there were no other women like them.

Although most of the women studied by Jensen (1999) had early clues about their same sex-gender orientation, they tended to stay in their marriages and tried to make them work. Six were married twenty or more years, ten between ten and twenty years, and the remaining eight stayed married from one to ten years. Nineteen of the women had children; most had two, one had three, one had four. Many enjoyed childbearing and child rearing and identified strongly with their roles as mothers.

Same sex-gender desires were so threatening to these women in terms of upsetting family, other relationships, the community, and their material well-being that they could not "let" themselves fully know about or act on these attractions. Even those aware of the optional path, did not feel free to determine their own path. Several women reported that they were not used to making decisions based on their own needs and desires and that they did not trust their own judgment. Many were blocked from fully knowing their attractions because of limited information and because of the pervasive heterosexist ideology. Positive same sex-gender relationship models were unavailable. Those who experienced same sex-gender relationships were all ultimately rejected by the other women. They did not perceive that a full relationship with a woman was a valid or available choice.

Another study (Charbonneau & Lander, 1991; Lander & Charbonneau, 1990) focused on thirty women who identified as lesbians in midlife. They were between the ages of thirty-five and fifty-five and were of varied ethnic, religious, and social backgrounds. Although most were of European ancestry, 20 percent were African American or Caribbean American. One-third grew up in working-class families, the others in middle- and upper-middle-class families. All these women accepted traditional definitions of the "proper" goals for women: marriage and motherhood. One never married but was engaged three times. The others had been married from one to thirty-two years; the average length was 12.3 years. More than half remained in their marriages ten years or longer but at the time of the survey, none of the women were still with their husbands. All but six were mothers and four of the six who had no children tried to conceive but were unsuccessful. Most of these women had two or three children; several had four to six children.

Prior to midlife, the women in this sample did not realize or acknowledge attraction to other women, and with few exceptions, never considered it a possibility. Those who fell in love with a woman or experienced sexual attraction to a woman in midlife were surprised. Even more surprising was their willingness to embrace the label *lesbian*. Some of the women felt that they had always been lesbians (Charbonneau & Lander, 1991; Lander & Charbonneau, 1990).

No single event precipitated this midlife identity shift. Instead, a combination of events provided the context for change or challenged these women to question their assumed heterosexuality. The political context many women were involved in most likely readied them for nonconformity. Twenty of the women participated in various kinds of political work ranging from mainstream activities such as voter registration drives to more radical activities such as antiwar demonstrations (Charbonneau & Lander, 1991).

Half the women made no specific reference to the women's movement when discussing their move from a heterosexual to a lesbian identity, nor were they feminists. The other half actively participated in the women's movement, this created a climate for asking questions and looking at oneself from a different perspective. This was achieved through experiences such as consciousness-raising groups or reading feminist books. Some women recalled books that were important to them, including details. For others, particular feminist events in a feminist environment such as a women's concert or an all-woman's weekend were the catalyst for embracing a lesbian identity (Charbonneau & Lander, 1991).

Other turning points included a parent's serious illness or death, or their own serious illness, after which they realized the transience of life and began a review of their lives; divorce or the moment they first thought of leaving a marriage, although half of the women were divorced for several or many years before they thought about a lesbian identity; time apart from men (or being celibate) which provided an opportunity to be independent and fulfill their own needs without men; changes in daily life such as moving, entering school, leaving or entering a job, joining a consciousness-raising group, or entering therapy; discovering that a friend, work colleague, or relative was lesbian; or experiencing erotic feelings for another woman. Once these women self-identified as lesbian it was essential for them to dispel negative stereotypes about lesbians. For some, this was a slow process but for others it happened because of a single encounter with another woman (Charbonneau & Lander, 1991).

Positive Effects of the Change in Sexual Identity

Because many women who identified as lesbians in midlife lived for so long as self-identified heterosexuals, the change in sexual identification resulted in a radical transformation and redirection. Some felt "for the first time I am me" (Charbonneau & Lander, 1991). Others, after living with men most of their adult lives, described the intimacy with other women at a depth they never before experienced or even imagined (McGrath, 1990). Sexual awakening with another woman usually led not only to redefinition of sexual identity, but also of gender. Behavior which before was viewed as masculine and unacceptable for women was reinterpreted as acceptable. These women become comfortable with a combination of roles previously defined as male or female.

Costs of the Change in Sexual Identity

Women who come out as lesbian in midlife experience two basic kinds of costs. The first involves the loss of a primary link with a man, which includes privileges, fantasies of being cared for by a man, and social support. Involvement with a woman will not, in most social contexts, gain the same respect and status as a link with a man (Cummerton, 1982; de Monteflores & Schultz, 1978; Groves & Ventura, 1983; Kirkpatrick, 1989b). The second cost involves the negative reactions these women experience when they disclose their lesbian self-identification (Lander & Charbonneau, 1990).

The midlife women studied by Jensen (1999) who embraced their lesbian or bisexual identity talked about losses but felt they went through a positive life change. They did not mention negatives such as having a stigmatized identity. Only one woman mentioned the loss of entitlements via heterosexual marriage or feeling sad about the ending of a marriage, a heterosexual life, or a home. The women did, however, experience fears: primarily being able to take care of themselves and their children alone.

Twenty-two women, ages forty-seven to sixty-three, were interviewed by P. E. Woolf (1998). Sixteen were white, the others a mixture of other racial/ethnic groups. All but one had a high school education or higher. Eighteen had a bachelor's degree or higher; eleven had a master's degree or higher. The women lived in a large metropolitan area in the Pacific Northwest. They had all come out at or after age forty (between the ages of forty and fifty-five). Besides changing their sexual identity, they felt they entered another culture with a distinct set of values, codes, and norms. They also had to "normalize" their attraction to women. Despite some difficulties, such as feeling confused and uncertain about the rules, they eventually acculturated to a lesbian identity. This required a paradigm shift from viewing lesbians as stigmatized to acceptable and even admirable persons to imitate. The most common theme was the development of female support networks prior to transition. All the women experienced at least one of a variety of transitional markers such as female bonding, obsession with another woman, dreams/fantasies, feminist archetypes, nonconformity, a death, economic instability, negative sex with men, celibacy, promiscuity, divorce, the influence of the feminist movement, empty nest syndrome, or trauma.

Some gay persons recognize their same sex-gender desires early in life and begin to follow that path. Others know they are gay but do not act on it until midlife. Men who know they are gay while married often struggled with guilt and secrecy; some have sexual encounters with other men while still married (Kimmel and Sang, 1995). Others report they were unaware of being gay until after divorce (Herdt et al., 1997).

Two ways of life for older lesbian and gay persons were identified by Cohler and Hostetler (2002). One group became aware of same sex-gender sexual wishes during childhood or adolescence. Typically they led a quiet life, often with partners. Their public and private lives were separated. They did not think of their sexual orientation as relevant to their work or in the community. Persons in the second group were mostly married and had adolescent or adult children, They had often not been aware of same sex-gender sexual desires until particular life circumstances occurred or because of increased visibility of LGB persons. Usually, they met another man or woman with whom they first experienced same sex-gender sexual desires. The first or a subsequent same sex-gender relationship led them to divorce and to establish a long-term relationship with their newly found same sex-gender partner (Herdt, 1997; Hostetler & Herdt, 1998; Ridge, Minichiello & Plummer, 1997).

Prior heterosexual marriage also made a significant difference for the lesbian and gay persons studied by Herdt et al. (1997), all of whom came out in midlife. A mostly white, well-educated, and professional sample completed a ten-month needs assessment study for older lesbian and gay persons in Chicago in 1996. The median age when the sample members identified as lesbian or gay was twenty-two; age twenty for gay persons and age thirty for lesbians. Those who married, however, tended to come out an average of ten years later than those who did not marry, usually after age thirty and for one-quarter of this group after age forty. The respondents differed in the degree to which they acknowledged their identity to themselves before divorce. Some always knew they were lesbian or gay or at least felt captivated by same sex-gender persons. Some reported illicit encounters with same sex-gender persons while still married. Other persons reported that they were not really cognizant of being lesbian or gay until after their divorce.

DISCLOSURES

Most coming-out models include sexual-identity disclosure to others as a necessary step in finalizing the identity development process. This step reinforces the post-Stonewall philosophy that hiding or staying in the closet perpetuates negative stereotypes, social oppression (D'Augelli & Garnets, 1995), and the idea that it is bad or wrong to be gay, lesbian, or bisexual (Healy, 1993; Herek, 1991). Disclosure of sexual identity has become easier (Hostetler, 2000), but LGB persons still hear negative comments from family and peers about LGB persons; they are well aware of what happens to some LGB persons who make disclosures (A. D. Martin, 1982). Openness can lead to rejection by family and friends and sometimes verbal and physical abuse (Hersch, 1988; A. D. Martin & Hetrick, 1988; Remafedi, 1987; Uribe & Harbeck, 1991). LGB persons can still lose child custody (e.g., Falk, 1989), jobs, and job promotions (e.g., M. Hall, 1989; M. P. Levine & Leonard, 1984).

Half of the midlife lesbians studied by Jensen (1999) feared losing custody of their children. Several delayed disclosure until their children were older to reduce the likelihood of a custody issue. At the least, a large majority of the women studied by Lander and Charbonneau (1990) experienced verbal harassment, such as being screamed at and being the recipient of painful comments. Many others experienced losses such as cancelled invitations to family occasions. These negative reactions were sobering because the women were previously unaware of the intensity of prejudice against LGB persons. Understandably, these kinds of reactions led many of these women to stop disclosing their sexual identity. Bradford and Ryan (1991) found many midlife lesbians in their sample were not open about their sexual identity with many individuals, including family members, heterosexual friends, and work associates.

In D'Augelli and Grossman's (2001) sample of older LGB persons (average age approximately seventy), the earliest disclosure was at age ten and the latest was at age sixty-eight. More than half had not told both parents about their sexual orientation and only 38 percent reported being known as LGB by more than three-quarters of their acquaintances. One-quarter was not known as LGB by co-workers; about half had not disclosed to employers. D'Augelli, Grossman, Hershberger, and O'Connell (2001) reported that approximately one-fifth of older lesbian and gay persons said less than 25 percent of their family of origin, children, co-workers (current and former), and employers (current and former) knew. The remaining 37 percent said more than 75 percent knew.

In a study on midlife gay persons, Schope (2002) collected data from 443 respondents (mean age of forty) who participated in various gay organizations in the Midwest. Most (91 percent) were white and 77 percent had a college degree. The respondents were placed into three groups:

1. Younger generation raised after Stonewall (ages sixteen to thirty)
2. Middle-age generation raised during the Stonewall era (ages thirty-one to forty-nine)
3. Older generation raised before Stonewall (ages fifty and over)

Two-thirds (63 percent) of the older generation had been completely closeted in school and 40 percent were currently closeted in their neighborhoods. They had developed strategies of secrecy to protect themselves from discrimination, and most likely these strategies were still in place. In contrast, those who grew up during and after Stonewall had less internalized oppression and were out significantly more in every setting. Rothblum et al. (1995) pointed out, however, that some midlife LGB persons do not live much differently from their counterparts in the 1940s and 1950s. This especially includes those who live in rural and conservative communities.

For many older lesbian and gay persons, the decision to not publicly identify their sexual identities allowed them to avoid the stressors of living in the highly oppressive pre-Stonewall culture. Older lesbian and gay persons came of age when living openly was extremely risky and dangerous. They could lose reputations, employment, housing, friends, and family. They could be arrested or put in mental hospitals (Fassinger, 1991; Claes & Moore, 2000). When disclosures were made to friends and families they were usually rejected, and often it was lifelong rejection. They also usually had no backup support networks of other lesbian and gay persons (Adelman, 1986).

Twenty African-American gay men age thirty-nine to seventy-three (average age of fifty-six), living in New York City, were interviewed by Adams and Kimmel (1997). Nearly all maintained ties with their biological families, but many had never discussed their sexual identification with their families. Many reported that when they first started experimenting sexually with other men, they limited themselves to white partners so that no one in the African-American community would detect their sexual identity. Six had been married, four had children; two others were not sure if they would have children or not. Twelve of the twenty were living alone at the time of the interview.

Sixty-two lesbians age fifty-five and older, living in Washington, Oregon, and California, were interviewed by T. C. Jones and Nystrom (2002). Over half (59 percent) were white. Ages ranged from fifty-five to ninety-five with a median age of sixty-five. Most of these women were educated beyond high school; 29 percent had some college; 21 percent a college degree; and 43 percent a graduate degree. Most (53 percent) of this group were retired; one-third (34 percent) were still employed. Household incomes ranged from under $10,000 to over $60,000, with the median income range of $30,000 to $39,000. Growing up in the 1940s and being part of the evolution of gay pride, most of these women believed that the gay rights movement had produced positive effects for younger lesbian and gay persons, but had little influence on their own lives. All of the women experienced a period of exploration, questioned their sexual identity, and tried to find safe situations in which to gather information about it. However, it was common for them to repress or suppress their sexual orientation. Some gave in to pressures to marry. Some who married denied their sexual identity and acknowledged it only after they were divorced and their children grown. Many reported that they currently tended not to be out or they were deliberate about whom they told about themselves. They reported high levels of life satisfaction.

One of the best-known organizations for older LGBT persons is SAGE (Senior Action in a Gay Environment) in New York City. Yet even many members of this organization are not out to the majority of persons in their lives. They do not feel safe opening up to health care and social work providers. They do not want their sexual identity to be an obstacle to receiving services. In coming-out groups at SAGE, with members ranging in age from forty to eighty, many gay men reported having loving marriages with women. They did not disclose their sexual identity to their wives because of the possibility of losing them, their children, and their jobs. Some, however, made disclosures soon after a divorce or the death of a spouse. Others came out after retirement when the fear of losing their livelihood no longer existed (Altman, 1999). Berger (1996) reported that as gay persons grow older, and especially as they retire, they have less reason to try to pass. They are less concerned about job loss and discrimination and generally more secure emotionally and financially. Some members of SAGE, however, still struggle to be true to themselves while living at home with a parent for whom they are caretakers (Altman, 1999).

Schneider (2002) reported on a seventy-five-year-old man who, after almost fifty years of marriage and after his wife and daughter had died, acknowledged he was gay. His wife knew but pretended his secret did not exist. His daughter never knew even as she was dying of cancer. The man said he did what society wanted him to do except he did see other men while married. When his wife found this out, however, she forbade him to do it again. He complied and did not have sex with another man until twenty-five years later.

In other studies, passing as heterosexual was not mentioned as a way of life although it was mentioned at specific times or in specific situations. Most older gay persons studied by L. B. Brown, Alley, Sarosy, Quarto, and Cook (2001) seemed to feel that others should accept them for the way they are, and they do not shy away from being openly gay. Perhaps historical changes since the 1960s have finally allowed gay persons to be more open with family and others. Berger and Kelly (2001) found that compared to younger gay persons, older gay persons worried less about exposure or cared less about who knew they were gay. They were more widely known to others as gay and less concerned about the opinions of parents and other relatives.

Now in retirement most of the gay persons studied by Hostetler, cited in Cohler & Galatzer (2000), were indifferent regarding disclosure of their sexual orientations. They did not go out of their way to tell others about their sexual identity and neither did they hide it. Those with partners led conventional and quiet social lives, and if they could afford it, hosted dinner parties for gay and heterosexual friends, went to the opera, theater, and concerts, and spent weekends and summers at vacation homes. With some exceptions, they did not believe that sexual identity had played a central role in their lives, and they were largely unaware of or indifferent to the events surrounding early gay liberation. Yet they acknowledged that social and political changes have made life easier for gay persons in general.

Although most of the older gay persons studied by Hostetler, cited in Cohler & Galatzer (2000), did not join in the gay rights movement, they were not hostile to it. In contrast, the older gay persons described in J. A. Lee's (1987) study were hostile toward the movement because they lost the status they had in the pre-Stonewall days. They resented the loss of this world and subculture, and the secret signs and rituals that they controlled. This world was adventuresome for them. Rosenfeld (2003) found that many of the older lesbian and gay persons in her sample felt pride in having passed as heterosexual. Lee's sample group did not like the pressure by gay liberationists for forced openness. Moreover, they found that the new liberated gay community rejected their attempts to join. Adelman's (1991) sample group of older lesbian and gay persons were frustrated and angered by the demands of secrecy on one hand and of disclosure on the other.

FAMILY OF ORIGIN

As the variable findings suggest, not all LGB persons have made many disclosures or at the very least, they have more difficulty with some audiences. The family of origin is first discussed followed by other family members, marital partners, and children. Disclosure to parents is the most difficult for LGB persons and probably evokes the greatest fear for children of any age. Disclosure of an older adult's LGB status can cause serious personal or family problems (D'Augelli & Grossman, 2001). Even today, the issue of a family member's sexual identity is often not discussed and rarely embraced. The relationships between older lesbian and gay persons and their families of origin are often maintained at a distance (Altman, 1999).

For those not ready to make disclosures to family, L. S. Brown (1989) identified several patterns of keeping one's sexual orientation hidden from the family. One pattern involves maintaining emotional and geographical distance from the family.

Another pattern, "I know you know," involves an unspoken agreement not to discuss a family member's sexual identification even though everyone knows it. This pattern might maintain stability in the family, but the cost is a lack of acknowledgment of one's life. The family will probably not acknowledge the partner or invite this person to family events. Another pattern, "Don't tell your father," involves an agreement that although disclosures are made to supportive siblings or mother, all agree not to tell other family members, especially father. Some LGB persons do not disclose to parents in order to avoid conflict or reprisal for themselves (Whittlin, 1983) and hurt or disappointment for their parents (Cain, 1991; D. Cramer & Roach, 1988). Many LGB persons, however, eventually disclose their sexual identities to their families because they feel uncomfortable or guilty about misleading them (e.g., Leaveck, 1994; Strommen, 1990). Or, they are unhappy with the impersonal distance between themselves and their families (e.g., L. S. Brown, 1989; D. Cramer & Roach, 1988). When children are at midlife, parents may not try to change them compared to trying to do this with younger or young adult children. Parents may recognize that their midlife child's sexual identity is not just a phase (Rothblum et al., 1995).

RACIAL AND ETHNIC FAMILIES

For most racial and ethnic lesbian and gay persons, the particular needs and values of their racial and ethnic groups present obstacles for identity development and disclosures (B. Smith, 1983). Most ethnic and racial persons feel strongly tied to their individual racial or ethnic communities because of oppression and the consequent need for group bonds (Kanuha, 1990). Their communities and extended families provide most of their social networks and support. Because the family provides the basic means of survival for the culture, family expectations take precedence over individual wishes (e.g., Chan, 1992; Wooden, Kawasaki, & Mayeda, 1983). Although the reactions of families to their lesbian and gay children may seem oppressive, the children may not be willing to risk the loss of support, affection, and security received from their families (Chan, 1992). Besides these common themes, unique issues also exist among different racial and ethnic groups (Rust, 1996a).

African-American Families

African-American lesbian and gay persons may hide their same sex-gender attractions from their families. This is largely because of the conservative Christian religiosity that dominates African-American communities (Bonilla & Porter, 1990; Greene, 1996). It claims that the Bible forbids same sex-gender sexual identities because they are a sin (Crisp, Priest, & Torgerson, 1998). Yet, in recent years, ambivalence, tolerance, and acceptance have emerged in African-American families (Manalansan, 1996; A. Smith, 1997). Survey data indicate that blacks are more supportive than whites of sexual orientation nondiscrimination laws (Yang, 1999). Family instructions such as "be silent and invisible" may allow the family to accept a lesbian, gay, or bisexual family member without having to deal with sexual orientation and the conflicts associated with it (Manalansan, 1996; A. Smith, 1997). As noted earlier, Adams and Kimmel (1997) found that most of the older gay black persons (average age fifty-six) they studied never specifically discussed their sexual identity with their families. This was the case although their families knew that they were gay. One exception was openness by some of these men with siblings.

Latino Families

Latino families are less outspoken about moral disapproval of same sex-gender sexual orientation than are African Americans families (Bonilla & Porter, 1990). They still maintain strong conservative attitudes, however, cultivated by Catholicism (Carballo-Digéuez,

1989; Rodriquez, 1996), so that disclosure of a gay or lesbian identity will likely meet with disapproval in these families (e.g., Espin, 1984, 1987; Morales, 1992). In addition, the Latino culture rigidly adheres to the traditions and practices of machismo and marianismo in the socialization of males and females. Males are supposed to become dominant and independent, characteristics of machismo, whereas females are supposed to model behaviors that manifest marianismo or represent the virtues of the Virgin Mary (Reyes, 1992). Increasingly, some Latino families are changing their attitudes toward LGB family members. This is due to dissimilarities in national origin, acculturation and assimilation statuses, socioeconomic status, educational level, and geographical residence. Resulting from increases in education, exposure to American culture, and the influence of feminism, a more equalitarian model is developing for Latino men and women (Marsiglia, 1998).

Asian-American Families

Asian-American families dictate the behavior and attitudes of their children (Savin-Williams, 1998b). They expect unquestioned obedience, and conformity (Chan, 1992) showed through respect and loyalty to parents and other elders (e.g., Liu and Chan, 1996; Lopez & Lam, 1998). Loyalty to siblings and one's marital partner follows in this order (Liu & Chan, 1996). The demand for conformity centers around expected sex-gender roles as rejection of these roles threatens the continuation of the family line (Chan, 1992; Wooden, Kawasaki, & Mayeda, 1983). Asian sons, who are the carriers of the family name, linkage, and heritage, are expected to marry and provide heirs (Chan, 1989), and care for older parents (Lopez & Lam, 1998). Women must fulfill the roles of dutiful daughter, wife, and mother (Chan, 1992). Same sex-gender sexual identity may be looked at as an act of treason against the family and the culture (Greene, 1997). Parents may refuse to discuss a disclosed lesbian or gay identity and may build a wall of silence between them and their child (Liu & Chan, 1996; Savin-Williams, 1996). Some Asian-American lesbian and gay persons, who more assimilated into Western culture, are more open about their sexual identity in non-Asian contexts (Chan, 1997; Nakajima, Chan, & Lee, 1996), but seldom with their parents (Chan, 1989).

The Vietnamese culture, following Confucian values, morally and socially condemns "homosexuality" (Nguyen, 1992). The fear of discovery becomes a source of mental pressure and anguish for lesbian and gay children from Vietnamese families (Lopez & Lam, 1998; Timberlake & Cook, 1984). Reactions to gay sons are particularly harsh as they are often abandoned by their families (Lopez & Lam, 1998),

Greek-American Families

Lesbian and gay children from Greek-American families often collude with their families' wishes to avoid conversations about same sex-gender sexual identities. Many Greek-American lesbian and gay persons, even if several generations removed from immigration, continue to identify strongly with their Greek heritage. Bonded by love and loyalty, the family maintains a link with the LGB child if disclosure is made, although it may be a superficial link (Fygetakis, 1997).

Native American Families

In contrast to other ethnic groups, traditional Native American families seldom disapprove of lesbian and gay daughters and sons (L. B. Brown, 1997) or pressure them to be other than who they are (M. A. Jacobs & Brown, 1997). Same sex-gender sexual orientation is just another form of difference in Native American cultures (L. B. Brown, 1997). Membership of Native Americans in a clan, an extended family, a tribe, or a nation lasts forever (Tofoya, 1996). L. B. Brown et al. (2001) reported that Native American gay persons they studied (mostly from ages fifty to age sixty-five) had regular contact with their families and that most families were aware of their sexual orientation. Nearly all reported being close, somewhat close, or very close to their families. Their sexual identity was acceptable to their families and to their Native American communities. Disclosures to their families caused no problems nor did they experience any discrimination within their communities.

Yet, and in contrast to other ethnic and racial groups, the attitudes of more acculturated Native Americans (third and fourth generations) are often more negative. This has resulted in large part from their adoption of Western Christian religions (K. L. Walters, 1997).

DISCLOSURES TO MARITAL PARTNERS

Most men who identify as bisexual while married soon tell their partners (M. S. Weinberg et al., 1994). Married gay persons, however, rarely disclose sexual identity out of fear of their wife and children's reactions, and their desire to preserve job security and social status (Strommen, 1989, 1990). Lesbian wives rarely make disclosures to marital partners because they fear their partners may react in a severe and angry manner, possibly with physical violence. Lesbian mothers fear custody battles, especially when their partners express extreme animosity toward them (Hanscombe and Forster, 1982).

Some lesbian and gay persons disclose to their marriage partners because of guilt about living a double life (Strommen, 1989). The early reactions of partners, largely based on indirect anecdotal accounts, may be similar to those of parents when their children make disclosures (e.g., Hanscombe & Forster, 1982; Kirkpatrick, Smith, & Roy, 1981). These reactions include: shock, estrangement, confusion, guilt, stigma, and sense of loss. They may feel that they were failures as wives or husbands (Gochros, 1985). A husband who discloses that he is HIV positive can cause a crisis and feelings of loss, betrayal, vulnerability, and uncertainty about the future (Paul, 1996).

Disclosure of a lesbian or gay sexual identity to a marital partner usually leads to divorce (Coleman, 1985a; Gochros, 1985). Wyers (1987) reported divorce rates as 97 percent for lesbian and 78 percent for gay persons. Divorce occurred for almost three-quarters of a sample of married gay persons studied by Scott and Ortiz (1996). Lesbian and bisexual women end marriages more quickly, because of a lack of sexual desire for the heterosexual partner, husbands' disparagement of their sexual identification, and a dislike of open marriages or secret extramarital relationships (Coleman, 1985a; Matteson, 1987). Sometimes the partners restructure their marital arrangements to adjust to a partner with a same sex-gender or bisexual sexual identity. They have an open or semi-open marriage or an "asexual" friendship with the marital partner (Gochros, 1989; Stokes & Damon, 1995; Whitney, 1990).

Studies on partnerships involving a transgender person are rare (Cole et al., 2000). Generally, the reaction of wives to the revelation of the partner's transgender identity is negative. They feel betrayed (Anderson, 1998; Emerson & Rosenfeld, 1996), used, abandoned, left out, and no longer needed (Hunt & Main, 1997). If a wife makes the discovery first, she may experience more intense feelings of betrayal and possibly will want to abandon the relationship. Because of rage about the discovery, she may disclose her husband's transgender identity to others (Cole et al., 2000).

One of the largest studies on women in relationships with transgender men was a six-year longitudinal study on 106 pairs. The men were predominantly cross-dressers. The women, who were members of informal discussion groups throughout the country, reported that the major obstacle to intimacy with their partners involved betrayal and lost trust. Yet, divorce was not prevalent; more than two-thirds of the wives never seriously thought about divorce or separation (G. R. Brown, 1998).

DISCLOSURES TO CHILDREN

Secrecy with children limits intimacy (Rohrbaugh, 1992), openness in addressing family issues (C. Patterson & Chan, 1997), and support (Matthews & Lease, 2000). Yet some lesbian and gay couples decide not to make disclosures of their sexual identity to their children (C. Patterson & Chan, 1997). It would involve a complex and delicate discussion of conception or why the child does not have a dad or a mom (Segal-Sklar, 1995). Many of these parents who do not live with or have custody of their biological children may also decide not to make disclosures to placate the custodial parent or members of the child's extended family who may control continued contact with the child (Appleby & Anastas, 1998). Openness can also result in harassment. Three-quarters of the lesbian and gay parents studied by Fredriksen (1999) had experienced harassment because of their sexual orientation: verbal (88 percent), emotional (50 percent), physical (9 percent), and sexual (9 percent).

If partners decide to disclose their sexual identities to children they have to decide when to do it, although the question of the best time to disclose to children remains unanswered. Generally, lesbian and gay parents should not tell children about their sexual identities until they are old enough to understand and ask questions. Parents should also feel confident about their sexual identities and sex-gender expressions before they make disclosures, and they should speak candidly about themselves and educate their children (Scasta, 1998).

Most lesbian and gay parents report that openness with their children improves their relationships in the long term (Hanscombe & Forster, 1982). Following disclosure of lesbian and gay parents, the reactions of children are usually positive (Bigner, 1996; Lott-Whitehead & Tully, 1993). They may respond with a sense of protectiveness toward their parents (O'Connell, 1993), or they may indicate that the information makes no difference or that they already knew it (Turner, Scadden, & Harris, 1990). This does not mean, however, that these children will have no more questions. Children often need continued discussions about the situation (C. J. Patterson, 1992). Gay fathers are not as open with their children as are lesbian mothers (Hanscombe & Forster, 1982). They fear that disclosure will damage their relationships with their children. However, children seldom reject their fathers because they are gay (Golombok, 2000).

In a study of bisexual men and women conducted by M. S. Weinberg et al. (1994), disclosures led to the positive outcomes of better communication and greater closeness between the parents and children. Some children, however, never talk with their parents about the disclosed knowledge and some find it difficult to explain bisexuality to their friends.

Relationships between transgender parents and their children are often strained because of the distance parents create to try to keep their children from discovering their identity. Whereas some of these parents may struggle with hiding existential issues such as identity and body image, those who cross-dress struggle with hiding clothing and makeup (Anderson, 1998). If they can keep their sex-gender expressions private, transgender parents sometimes decide to wait until all the children are older before disclosing their sex-gender desires. Some decide to be open so that all the family, including the partner, can develop understanding and coping skills together (Cole et al., 2000).

Children who accept their gay and lesbian parents are usually younger and often unaware of the stigma associated with being lesbian or gay (C. J. Patterson, 1992). Children first told of their parent's sexual identity in early adolescence might have a more difficult time adjusting than either younger or older children. Adolescence is when it is common for children to devalue parents in their struggle to carve out a separate identity. In addition, they typically conform to peer attitudes that may be hostile to same sex-gender sexual orientation or they may fear embarrassment and ridicule (Kirkparick, 1989a). Initially, they may react with distress, anxiety, anger, and sorrow, and may make deprecating statements to the parents (Appleby & Anastas, 1998). Particularly, male adolescents who are trying to assert masculine characteristics can be deeply troubled by a parent's announcement of a same sex-gender sexual orientation (Scasta, 1998). Mothers may experience devaluation and discrimination against lesbian and gay persons so dealing with adolescent children might be especially painful (Kirkpatrick, 1989a). Relationships with adolescent children can also be difficult for mothers just coming out as lesbians at midlife (Kirkpatrick, 1988,1989a; Rothschild, 1991; Sang, 1992a). Midlife and older lesbians studied by T. C. Jones and Nystrom (2002) who disclosed to their children reported that many of their reactions were supportive. Some of the children, however, expressed confusion, resentment, anger, fear of their friends' responses, and questions about their own sexuality. If there were two or more children in a family, it was common for each of them to express different emotions.

Older adolescents who came from heterosexual marriages and now live with lesbian or gay parents may suddenly worry about being seen as different by their peers (Hargaden & Llewellin, 1996) and may fear being stigmatized or rejected (Rothschild, 1991). Peers may taunt them (Sears, 1993-1994) or harm them in other ways (Scasta, 1998). These children may not tell anyone about their family situation because they do not want to risk being singled out; they may not even bring friends and dates home (Matthews & Lease, 2000).

D. Cramer (1986) reported that younger children of lesbian mothers rarely recall harassment from peers. Other studies reported that younger children are just as popular and have no more difficulty making friends than do younger children with heterosexual parents (Golombok, Spencer, & Rutter, 1983). Adolescent children are more likely to receive negative messages from peers about their parents' sexual orientation (Matthews & Lease, 2000). Other researchers have reported, however, that although incidents of peer group teasing have been recorded, relationships with peers are generally good (Tasker & Golombok, 1997). Even so, a support group for children of lesbian or gay parents can provide stress relief and friendships of others in similar situations.

Parents should help children decide whom to tell. To avoid harassment, children should use discretion in disclosures. Parents may need to intervene in school and other arenas if harassment does occur

(Scasta, 1998); however, some parents may caution their children not to disclose their sexual orientation and the children may feel the same. The secrecy about disclosure, however, can create anxiety for the both parents and children (Crawford, 1987).

Some lesbian or gay parents are still working on their own identity issues. Children who tell others may "out" lesbian or gay parents to extended family members and society at large. This can provoke anxiety (Rothberg & Weinstein, 1996), and if involved in custody battles, can also strain couples (Rutter & Schwartz, 1996). Parents need to develop constructive coping mechanisms for themselves and for helping their children cope with stress and other challenges (Baum, 1996; Bigner, 1996).

Parents also make decisions regarding disclosures to a variety of persons involved in a child's life such as medical staff, child care workers, and school officials. For instance, are they going to cross out "father" or "mother" on forms and put in "other mother" or "other father" or "parent-parent" (Segal-Sklar, 1995). More than half (51 percent) of the lesbian and gay parents studied by Fredriksen (1999) were out to all co-workers, 58 percent to medical services providers, 65 percent to school personnel, and 34 percent to neighbors. Parents must also make decisions about how to handle ordinary encounters and questions when out in the world such as walking in a park or shopping in a grocery store (A. Martin, 1993).

DISCLOSURE MANAGEMENT

LGBT persons constantly weigh when and where to disclose, to whom, and the possible consequences (A. S. Walters & Phillips, 1994). Some persons may disclose to co-workers at a particular job but revert to the closet if they change jobs, or if they move from a large city to a small town (Cruikshank, 1992). In late life, persons may decide to close the door on the closet, perhaps forever, if they enter a predominantly heterosexual and likely heterosexist nursing home. A cost-benefit analysis can be used to determine whether to make disclosures (Cain, 1991). Gonsiorek (1993) recommended the concept of rational "outness" or being as open as possible but closed if necessary to protect oneself from discrimination.

SUMMARY

   Coming out is the internal process of recognizing that one is lesbian, gay, bisexual, or transgender. Models for coming out describe
the process in stages, but not everyone follows a smooth sequence of
steps or gets to the end of the process, which in most models includes
public disclosures and political activism. Most coming-out models
are also dated and have numerous gaps such as the effects of race and
ethnicity, social class, historical contexts, and sex-gender. Not everyone makes sexual-identity disclosures and often, only to selected audiences such as siblings but not parents. Others such as racial and ethnic persons face more obstacles in making disclosures because of
cultural and religious beliefs. Disclosure to parents is likely the most
difficult for any LGBT person.

PART II:
LIFE ARENAS

Chapter 3

Education, Work, Income, and Community Participation

EDUCATION AND INCOME

Studies of educational attainment of midlife lesbians found that most of the respondents completed higher education programs. Among the Bradford and Ryan (1991) respondents, only a small number (15 percent) attained no college education. About one-quarter (24 percent) graduated from college or completed some graduate work, and almost half (48 percent) completed a graduate or professional degree. The midlife lesbians studied by Sang (1990, 1991, 1992a, 1992b, 1993) were also a highly educated group. Only a few (6 percent) stopped their education after graduating from high school. Some held bachelor's degrees (12 percent), but a larger group held master's degrees or more than a bachelor's degree (45 percent), or doctorate degrees (24 percent).

In the Chicago sample of 160 older lesbian and gay persons studied by Beeler et al. (1999) and Herdt et al. (1997), 31 percent held bachelor's degrees, 58 percent graduate or professional degrees. In their sample of sixty-two older lesbians, T. C. Jones and Nystrom (2002) found that a significant proportion (64 percent) obtained college or graduate degrees. Most (65 percent) older lesbian and gay persons studied by Grossman et al. (2001) had bachelor's or higher degrees, 14 percent associate degrees or certificates of various types, 21 percent high school diplomas. Yearly income ranged from $15,000 (15 percent), $15,000 to $35,000 (44 percent), to more than $35,000 (41 percent). Most gay men (ages fifty to sixty-five) studied by L. B. Brown et al., 2001) were highly educated, ranging from some college to postgraduate work. Incomes ranged from $20,000 a year to $70,000. D. Rosenfeld (2003) interviewed twenty-five gay and twenty-five lesbian persons in Los Angeles. They ranged in age from sixty-four to eighty-nine (average age seventy-three years). More than one-third (37 percent) were seventy-five or older, 14 percent eighty or older. Annual income ranged from below $10,000 to more than $100,000 (average for gay men $29,500, for lesbians $24,700). Butler and Hope (1999) studied a sample of twenty-one lesbians, age fifty-four to seventy-four (mean of fifty-nine) living in Maine. They had a mean income of $23,000. The range was from considerable wealth to no income.

WORK ASPIRATIONS AND WORK LIVES

Most older lesbian and gay persons are retired. For example, three-quarters (74 percent) of the older lesbian and gay persons (mean age: sixty-eight) studied by Grossman et al. (2001) were retired, 18 percent working; 5 percent were working past retirement.

For many midlife gay persons, their stage of life is the same as for heterosexual men in that they focus on occupational achievements and establishing connections with friends and a special partner (Kimmel & Sang, 1995; Vaillant, 1977). The career ladders of gay men, however, may differ from those of heterosexual men because of discrimination due to sexual orientation, if known. If not known, gay men may have to make continual efforts to hide their sexual orientation.

As they begin to ascend work hierarchies, gay employees may resist identities as "company men" to avoid discovery of their sexual orientation ("Homosexuals Said to Face," 1994). Or they may be hindered from moving up the ladder in the corporate world because of their single status or appearance as such. Not being an established "family man" can be an obstacle to career development and advancement (Hostetler, 2000). Some gay persons do not pursue higher level positions because they desire more balance between their career and their personal life (Kimmel & Sang, 1995).

For those concerned about discovery of their sexual orientation and discrimination, self-employment can be an answer (M. S. Weinberg & Williams, 1974; Berger, 1996). Leaders in lesbian and gay communities are often self-employed (Russo, 1982).

Some older gay men interviewed by Hostetler (2000) worked in gay-identified jobs, such as hairdressing and interior design, and generally had supportive co-workers. Others worked in low-profile positions as librarians, government bureaucrats, and engineers, and although they were not necessarily out at work, they experienced little tension regarding their sexual orientation.

Most lesbians have been financially independent and have worked during their adult lives. Most are following the linear career pattern having started this path, on average, at twenty-six years of age. For those who came out earlier, self-support began in the early twenties (Fertitta, 1984; Sang, 1991). Others followed paths similar to those of heterosexual women by seeking new directions after their children were older (Faderman, 1991). Many older lesbians studied by T. C. Jones and Nystrom (2002) were also mostly self-sufficient and financially independent for the majority of their lives. Some started working in their teens; some are still working in their seventies and eighties. They reported that self-esteem was often entwined with their accomplishments in the workplace. Many also reported a great sense of personal satisfaction from success at work and being able to raise their children successfully, often on their own.

Early studies of heterosexual midlife women indicated that they were inclined to form dreams in their teens and twenties that placed them in adulthood as wives and supporters of their husbands' goals. They had few dreams in which occupation was the primary component (Roberts & Newton, 1987). The scenario differed for midlife lesbians. For example, lesbians studied by Sang (1990), who never married were highly likely to project career goals for themselves (78 percent), probably because they had to depend on themselves for economic support. In adolescence, they had dreams of career and adventure. Those who identified as lesbian in their teens and twenties were more likely to have career expectations early, compared to those who identified as lesbian in their thirties or when they were over forty. They also tended to be nontraditional during adolescence such as being athletic or bookish. They were more likely to envision themselves in nontraditional careers such as science, medicine, or business.

The life dreams that midlife lesbians reported having in adolescence were placed by Sang (1990) in one of three categories: "Relational Life Dreams (marriage and family only or no life dreams), . . . Traditional and Non-Traditional Life Dreams (career plus family), [and] Non-Traditional Life Dreams (career, work, travel, adventure, impact on the world—no mention of marriage and family)" (p. 114). Midlife lesbians who were more likely to hold nontraditional life dreams in adolescence (careers, no marriage) identified themselves as lesbian in their teens and twenties. Those who identified as lesbian in their thirties or in midlife reported dreams that were equally divided among all three life dream categories.

Although just a little more than half of the midlife lesbians in Sang's (1990) sample expected to hold careers as adults, almost all were in careers. More than three-fourths of these women were professionals while the others were in business or held working-class jobs. Half of the women were in nontraditional careers or jobs for women such as university dean, financial analyst, and truck driver. Almost all the midlife lesbian respondents studied by Bradford and Ryan (1991) worked. Compared with employed women in this age group in the general population, midlife lesbians were four times as likely to work in professional or technical fields. More often than not, the women in this sample worked as managers or administrators. Others worked as clerical workers, craftswomen, service workers, and skilled and unskilled laborers. Faderman (1991) observed that some lesbians pursue low-paying jobs or are unemployed or underemployed while active in grassroots politics.

Most of the women who identified as lesbian after age forty envisioned themselves in traditional careers such as nursing and teaching (Sang, 1990). Women not out as lesbians until midlife were also more similar to traditional heterosexual women in that primary relationships (61 percent) were more important to them than work (21 percent). If in a new, novel, and exciting relationship they may place more importance on the relationship than on work. This does not mean, however, that they are not committed to and satisfied with their work (Sang, 1992b).

As they get older, lesbians who worked all of their adult lives may want to work in a different way such as spending fewer hours at work or making career changes (Sang, 1992b). Among the overriding desires for some midlife lesbians may be to have more balance between work commitments and personal endeavors ("Homosexuals Said to Face," 1994).

COMMUNITY DEVELOPMENT AND PARTICIPATION

Rather than return to their hometowns at the end of World War II, men and women who came to identify as "homosexual" while in the armed forces often remained in the port cities where they disembarked after the war. This included cities such as New York, Los Angeles, Baltimore, San Francisco, Boston, New Orleans, Seattle, and Washington, DC. "Homosexual" subculture subsequently thrived in these cities (Berubé, 1990). Individuals residing in these port cities organized social and political groups including the East Coast Homophile Organization (ECHO) founded by Dr. Frank Kameny in Washington, DC, in 1963; the Mattachine Society founded by Harry Hay in Los Angeles in 1950 for gay persons, and the first "gay rights" group in the United States; and the Daughters of Bilitis founded by Del Martin and Phyllis Lyon in San Francisco in 1955 for lesbians (D'Emilio, 1983; D. Martin & Lyon, 1995; Schultz, 2001). Given the times, these organizations were courageous in their efforts to challenge discrimination against "homosexuals." These groups thought that discrimination and prejudice resulted from misinformation about "homosexuals" as different if not dangerous, and they tried to educate the public that they were no different from heterosexuals (Seidman, 2002). They dressed and acted in accordance with mainstream standards and avoided overt displays of their sexual identities. Their attempts to fit in with mainstream society, however, did not achieve social acceptance (Bohan, 1996). A national conference held in Denver in 1959 by the Mattachine Society was reported in the *Denver Post*. The local organizer was arrested and jailed for sixty days. His home was searched, and he lost his job. It was not until a U.S. Supreme Court ruling in January 1958 that lesbian and gay publications such as the *Mattachine Review* could be delivered by the post office. Before this time, these publications were considered obscene (Loughery, 1998).

Persons in some settings in the 1950s were unconcerned with approval or acceptance by mainstream society. This included lesbians in Buffalo, New York, described by Kennedy and Davis (1993). These women often went to bars and parties, and experienced solidarity and feelings of pride. They lived independent and nonconformist lives by crossing acceptable boundaries for women, as in avoiding marriage to men and living with women. These lesbians and the members of the Mattachine Society and other early groups were the beginnings of community for lesbian and gay persons. Aside from gravitation of lesbian and gay persons to large urban cities where others like them are concentrated, lesbian and gay residential areas exist in some large cities, such as the Castro in San Francisco, West Hollywood in Los Angeles, New Town in Chicago, Coconut Grove in Miami, and Greenwich Village in New York. Even in smaller cities, lesbian and gay persons tend to live close to one another (D'Emilio, 1993; Nakayama & Corey, 1993; M. Pope, 1995).

In rural areas and suburbs, a small lesbian or gay bar may still provide the only way to have face-to-face contact. But, many national and international organizations and a multitude of Internet lists and Web sites also connect LGBT persons throughout the world. This means to connect with each other is especially useful for those who live in small towns, small cities, and rural areas (D'Augelli & Garnets, 1995; Miller, 1990).

Lesbian and gay newspapers, magazines, and Web sites advertise groups and activities open to new members, usually in large urban areas. Lesbian and gay yellow pages and Lambda pages also list numerous organizations and resources as well as places to meet. Most large cities also have Parents, Families and Friends of Lesbians and Gays (PFLAG) groups open to anyone interested in affirmative actions on behalf of families with LGBT children of any age. PFLAG is an international organization represented in 444 communities across the United States and in eleven other countries (D'Augelli & Garnets, 1995; F. R. Lynch, 1992).

Groups for bisexual men and women now exist in almost every state in the United States and in many other countries. This includes the national bisexual political and educational organization BiNet USA, which developed in 1992 out of the North American Bisexual Network that was established in 1990. An international network of various bisexual groups including support groups and political action groups is also available. An identifiable bisexual press and forum exist for debates on bisexual political ideology (Hutchins, 1996; Rust, 1995). In addition, today cable television shows, college courses, Web sites, and e-mail lists address bisexual topics. *The Bisexual Resource Guide* (Ochs, 2001) provides lists of bisexual organizations throughout the world and other information such as bibliographies and filmographies.

Transgender persons who are out usually desire to contribute to the development of other transgender persons through being visible and providing support groups and newsletters. Online computer forums publish autobiographies that introduce newcomers to the community (Nakamura, 1997). To find another transgender person is a tremendous emotional and psychological relief (Gagné & Tewksbury, 1999). The magazine *Transgender* provides news, views, and features for the transgender community and friends. The number of books in print on transgender issues is increasing daily (Maurer, 1999).

Community Participation

Midlife Persons

All the midlife lesbians studied by T. C. Jones and Nystrom (2002) were actively involved with support systems that included family, partners, friends, community groups, and religious/spiritual affiliations. Three-fourths of the Bradford and Ryan (1991) sample of midlife lesbians lived in communities with at least a few lesbian-related activities or support services. Most had access to activities specifically for lesbians and most regularly attended events for only lesbians. Attendance at these events was once or twice a month for about half of the sample (52 percent), once a week (16 percent), to less than once a year (6 percent). The most frequent activities were supportive, social, or lesbian and gay rights oriented. More than one-third (37 percent) participated in lesbian and gay rights organizations. These participants were more likely to be open about their sexual identities.

Participation of midlife lesbians in general community activities was more limited. The most involvement (about 33 percent) was with union or professional group meetings, 22 percent political groups, 18 percent health centers or clubs, 14 percent minority political groups (not specifically focused on lesbians and gay persons), 13 percent neighborhood associations, and 10 percent groups related to children's needs (Bradford & Ryan, 1991). In Woodman's (1987) study of lesbian and gay organizations, she found fewer midlife lesbians affiliated with community resources (34 percent). Often, midlife lesbians felt in a bind. They feared both disclosure of their sexual orientation and social isolation from others who might be potential friends. Two-thirds (64 percent) of the women in this sample were from the Southwest, South, and Midwest which likely played some part in inhibiting participation in community activities.

Older Persons

Most of the older gay persons studied by L. B. Brown et al. (2001) reported being involved with the gay community in some capacity, while about 15 percent had no involvement. Most viewed gay bars, nightclubs, and beaches as necessary places to build camaraderie and community.

The older lesbian and gay persons in Berger's (1984) study actively participated in both the lesbian and gay community and heterosexual community. Most of the older lesbians and gay persons studied by Minnigerode and Adelman (1978) participated in social and political organizations. Quam and Whitford (1992) reported high involvement of older lesbians and gay persons in their communities. In Grossman et al.'s (2001) national sample of 416 LGB adults (age range: 60-91, average age 68.5), more than three-fourths (79 percent) were members of gay-identified agencies or groups. About half (51 percent) reported belonging to one or two gay or lesbian organizations, others reported up to twenty groups. Most (66 percent) said they attend one or two groups regularly. Some indicated attending no groups regularly, others up to eight groups regularly. Some attended no groups at all. Many older lesbian and gay persons studied by D'Augelli et al. (2001) reported weekly contact with other LGB persons (59 percent), with one-quarter reporting that they had daily contact. Most (91 percent) indicated that they were members in one to twenty gay/lesbian organizations. In a sample of older lesbian and gay persons studied by Beeler et al. (1999), 59 percent were moderately or exceedingly involved with the lesbian and gay community. Of the women, however, 48 percent were not very involved and only 19 percent exceedingly involved. Only 8 percent of women over age fifty-one were exceedingly involved. More gay men (69 percent) than lesbians (27 percent) went to bars. Sixty-one percent of the whole sample spent time with younger LGB persons, often participating in sports, church, or social activities. This might include seventy-year-olds with forty-year-olds. Most of the older gay men studied by Kertzner (1999) described frequent and meaningful social interactions with peers (less frequently younger adults) through volunteerism, participation in recreational or support groups, or work-related activities. The respondents were divided in opinion about the importance and rewards of socializing with younger adults and particularly with younger gay persons; no single pattern of intergenerational socialization characterized the sample. Lesbian communities are less stratified by age than gay communities. Lesbians of different ages see themselves as peers (Rothblum et al., 1995). Kehoe (1989) also reported that lesbians of various ages participated in the same social and political events.

The specific types of community involvement of older lesbian and gay respondents was studied by Quam and Whitford (1992) as well as other researchers:

1. *Bars:* Over the past two months prior to the study by Quam and Whitford (1992), men (47.5 percent) were significantly more likely to visit a bar than women (23.1 percent). This included 35 percent for all participants. Gray and Dressel (1985) found that older gay men did not visit bars as often as younger gay men. They tended, instead, to participate more in parties with private groups of friends. Although many older gay men studied by L. B. Brown et al. (2001) reported going to gay bars, they also reported feeling out of place because of age.

2. *Social organizations:* Two-thirds of the Quam and Whitford (1992) sample participated in social groups. Lesbians (77 percent) were more likely to participate than gay men (52.5 percent). The large majority (80 percent) would consider participating in a lesbian or gay social organization, eventually. Most older lesbians were interested (92.3 percent) compared to 65 percent of gay men. If the organization included both lesbians and gay persons, more than three-quarters (78.8 percent) of the total sample would still be interested. They were much less interested (33.8 percent) in a social organization for older women or older men that included heterosexuals. Even less (27 percent) would consider participating in a general population social organization. Very few (8.8 percent) actually participated in a general population senior center or club. Gay men (40 percent) expressed greater interest in this type of organization. Quam (1993) suggested that a general population social organization for older persons did not offer the safety found in lesbian and gay organizations. Also, the chances were much better in a lesbian and gay social organization to meet potential friends and partners. Gay men complained that they were often pursued by older heterosexual women in general population organizations.

3. *Social service, political, religious, senior services:* For the total group studied by Quam and Whitford (1992), participation was relatively low in social service organizations such as community action groups or AIDS services (22.5 percent) and political organizations (11.3 percent). It was higher in religious organizations (33.8 percent) with a significant difference between those over sixty (20 percent) and under sixty (43 percent). Most older lesbians were raised within a religious context but many moved away from organized religion (Minnigerode & Adelman, 1978; Tully, 1983). Church attendance was not frequent for older lesbians studied by Kehoe (1986), and 60 percent claimed no religious affiliation. In a study of older lesbians, Tully (1992) found that religious and formal educational institutions were not viewed as sources of support.

As noted, some older lesbian and gay persons have never participated in the community. In their sample of old-old lesbian and gay persons (aged seventy-five to ninety), Quam and Whitford (1992) found that they were unlikely to participate in community services most likely because they wanted to continue concealing their sexual orientation. In contrast, the young-old cohort (aged sixty to seventy-five or eighty) seemed quite interested in pertinent services and programs. L. B. Brown et al. (1997) generally found that gay persons with a mean age of sixty-three involved themselves in various activities in the gay community. Berger and Kelly (2001) reported that compared with younger gay men, older gay men participate less often in the public gay community (bars, social and political clubs, etc.). They rely more heavily on long-standing friendship networks. When they do seek involvement outside the home, they more likely participate in religious activities and social service organizations. Participation in social and political activities decreased as they aged (e.g., Berger, 1996).

Friend (1990) found that older lesbian and gay members of his affirmative group were more likely to use resources of the lesbian and gay community. An executive director of SAGE, Dawson (1982) indicated that the largest percentage of older adults with whom he worked was vibrant, active, and independent. For other older lesbian and gay persons who were not affirmative (Friend, 1990), it was more difficult for them to develop a place in the modern lesbian and gay community. Some wanted contact with other lesbian and gay persons but with no disclosure of their private lives. There was likely to be tension between these persons and more public and politically active persons (Lee, 1989). Friend (1990) thought that members of the "passing" group who used social service programs would seek more traditional senior centers and not those focused on lesbian and gay persons. Those in the isolated "stereotypic" group would likely not seek services even in traditional centers.

BENEFITS OF COMMUNITY INVOLVEMENT

Integration into the lesbian and gay community is important, especially when family ties are weak or missing (Raphael & Robinson, 1980; Wolf, 1978). Even when family support exists, it is fortified by support from friends (Friend, 1980; Raphael & Robinson, 1980) and community. Adelman (1991) found that high life satisfaction was related to low community involvement for older lesbian and gay persons. However, other studies found that older lesbian and gay persons experienced positive results from being integrated into the lesbian and gay community through social, political, or religious activities. Older gay men were less fearful of aging, more self-accepting, less-depressed (Berger, 1996); higher in self-esteem, self-worth, and psychological well-being (M. S. Weinberg & Williams, 1974); and were happier (J. A. Lee, 1987). Linkage to the lesbian community was important in Fertitta's (1984) study for self-acceptance and a positive lesbian identity. Almost all sixty-eight participants in that study were involved in the lesbian community. Lesbian and gay persons who participate in political and social activities within the lesbian and gay community report less impact of heterosexism on morale than those who are less involved (Hostetler, 2000). Older lesbian and gay persons who were active in service and political organizations were more likely to believe that their sexual orientation did not hinder adjustment to aging, whereas the opposite resulted for those who were inactive in these organizations (Quam & Whitford, 1992). One study showed different outcomes by age groups. For example, participation in social and religious organizations contributed to life satisfaction for younger gay persons (ages fifty to fifty-nine), but did not make this difference for those age sixty and older (Quam & Whitford, 1992; Whitford, 1997).

SOCIAL SERVICES

As GLBT persons grow older, they enter a service world that may not be familiar to them. Some activists have created GLBT-specific organizations, such as Senior Action in a Gay Environment (SAGE). These types of organizations are not available in all parts of the country and cannot provide all needed services, but older lesbian and gay organizations are growing in the United States and Canada (Friend, 1987). Founded in 1977, SAGE is the most successful and enduring of the organizations. It is a model program which provides advocacy, policy leadership, and direct services in an intergenerational context (Cahill et al., 2000). It provides regular visits by "friendly visitors" and "telephone reassurance" or regular phone calls for homebound persons. Social events are scheduled monthly such as dinners, dances, and discussion groups (Gwenwald, 1984).

Not many cities offer any equivalent to SAGE. However, for more than twenty years SAGE has worked to train other communities to develop similar organizations. For example, SAGE programs are now in place in Connecticut, Florida, Illinois, Massachusetts, Michigan, Minnesota, Nebraska, New York, Oregon, Rhode Island, Wisconsin, and Ontario (Canada) (SAGE, 2001). The LA Gay & Lesbian Center sponsors a senior program that provides similar services. New Leaf Outreach to Elders (formerly GLOE) in San Francisco also provides similar services (Reid, 1995). For example, this group is dedicated to helping older adults foster friendships, visiting homebound seniors, and building community. It offers a variety of support groups, discussion groups, social meetings, seminars, and a friendly visiting program that trains volunteers to work with older adults. New Leaf encourages the goals of another nonprofit organization, Rainbow Adult Community Housing (RACH), which are to help build an intergenerational LGBT community, and a facility to house this community (Blando, 2001).

Other services are not comprehensive compared to these programs. Prime Timers is a self-help group started in Boston but available in other parts of the country (McDougall, 1993). Grior Circle organizes African-Amercian GLBT elders in the New York City area. Old Lesbians Organizing for Change (OLOC) has made efforts to bridge the gap between academics and activists who advocate on behalf of older lesbians. Red Dot Girls in Seattle, Washington, is a model community-building project for older lesbians. Pride Senior Network advocates for the needs of GLBT elders in New York City and New York State. The International Longitudinal Transsexual and Transgender Aging Institute in Richmond, Virginia, researches, publishes, and supports the needs of transgender elders (Cahill et al., 2000).

SUMMARY

Most lesbian and gay persons have worked all their adult lives and many in the samples studied completed a higher education program including master's and doctoral degrees. Gay men who do not want others to know their sexual identity may not seek career advancement if it includes higher visibility or they are not considered for advancement because they are not seen as "family men." Some choose to work in gay-identified businesses such as interior design or low-profile positions such as librarians. Many lesbians are or have been career oriented, and the earlier they came out the more likely they were to hold nontraditional careers for women. Community development expanded after World War II, especially in cities where lesbian and gay persons in the military disembarked when the war was over. It is still the case that community activities are more available in large urban cities than in suburbs, small towns, or rural areas. Bisexual and transgender persons have also developed group activities. Most midlife and older lesbian and gay persons participate to some degree in community activities, although for some the obstacle of not wanting to be out still operates. Most studies report a multitude of benefits resulting from community participation.

Chapter 4

Family Links

Midlife and older LGBT persons are not different from the same population of heterosexual persons in terms of family of origin, friends, partners, and in many instances children (Kimmel, 1992). Although the data are limited, these family statuses are addressed here.

OLDER PARENT-CHILD LINKS

Few studies have focused on midlife or older lesbian and gay persons and their parents. T. C. Jones and Nystrom (2002) in their study of older lesbians found that partners were their primary relationships, with friends and biological family members following. All acknowledged an emotional link to their biological families although some were estranged from them. Parental relationships were often mixes of friction and harmony. Some of the women indicated that they never came out to their parents or that, when they did, their parents refused to discuss the subject. However, many reported that family members became more accepting of their sexual orientation and their partners over time. L. B. Brown et al. (2001), in a study of sixty-nine gay persons, ages thirty-six to seventy-nine (mostly fifty to sixty-five), found that most were in regular contact with their families and that their families were aware of their sexual orientation.

One rare study by Warshow (1991) focused on the links between mothers and midlife lesbian daughters. The sample included twenty daughters between the ages of forty and fifty-seven living in New York City. All the respondents were middle class and well educated (two-thirds completed graduate degrees); all except two were white. They varied in their acceptance of a lesbian identity: nonaccepting (two), defensively accepting (eight), accepting (private) (six), and accepting (political) (four). The mother-daughter links were described as unchanged negative (eight), changed from negative to positive (seven), unchanged positive (three), and idealization of mothers with no conscious negative feelings about them at any time (two).

Eight of the ten daughters with the most negative feelings about their sexual orientation (nonaccepting and defensively accepting) experienced consistently negative links with their mothers. The links with mothers for seven of the ten daughters with the most positive feelings about their sexual orientation (accepting private and accepting political) changed from negative to positive. Working out their own self-acceptance was a prerequisite for daughters to have more satisfactory links with their mothers. It was important for them to experience a period of creating strong identities as lesbians. They also needed to integrate other interests and persons into their lives. This helped to counteract negativism about their identities, and only after this happened did many of these women reevaluate their relationships with their mothers (Warshow, 1991).

Some of the mothers studied by Warshow (1991) were physically and/or emotionally abusive to their daughters. In these situations, the daughters first had to work through the abuse before dealing with the rejection of their sexual orientation. Other mothers were self-sacrificing, which seemed to make it difficult for the daughters to differentiate from them and find their own path in life. These mothers expected their daughters in turn to be self-sacrificing on behalf of their mothers. Other mothers experienced pleasure in their daughters' development. They did not pressure them to agree with their ideas of right and wrong.

SPECIAL ROLES IN ONE'S FAMILY OF ORIGIN

Some lesbian and gay persons who interact with their families of origin carry out special roles such as providing financial assistance, counseling support, and aid in times of crisis (Kimmel, 1992). Sometimes they are selected as the caregiver of an aging parent or other relative. One out of three lesbian and gay persons provides some kind of caregiving assistance either to children or adults with an illness or disability (Fredriksen, 1999). In a sample of African-American lesbian and gay persons, aging parents were more likely to reside in the home of immediate family and less likely to enter a nursing home compared to aging parents of other ethnic backgrounds (Mays, Chatters, Cochran, & Mackness, 1998).

Lesbian and gay children might be selected for caregiving because they are unmarried and may seem more geographically mobile. LGBT persons, however, are not always happy with this responsibility. In focus groups done by the National Gay and Lesbian Task Force (NGLTF) Policy Institute and Pride Senior Network with older LGBT persons across New York City in 2000, many persons reported frustration and resentment at heterosexual siblings who look to them to provide primary care for ailing elderly parents. They were viewed as "single" while heterosexual siblings were presumed busy with a married partner and children (cited in Cahill et al., 2000, p. 112). Although an extensive amount of literature exists on caregiving for older family members, little of it focuses on the experiences of lesbian and gay caregivers. Fredriksen (1999) provided a rare report, but only on the demographics of 1,466 lesbian and gay persons with adult care responsibilities. Approximately 40 percent were between ages thirty and thirty-nine, and slightly more than one-quarter (26 percent) were between ages forty and forty-nine. Lesbians with adult care responsibilities were significantly more likely to be older and less educated and more likely to be partnered than lesbians without such responsibilities. Gay caregivers of adults, compared with those who did not provide such caregiving, were significantly more likely to be unemployed and older. Lesbian caregivers were significantly more likely to have a partner than gay caregivers (69 percent of lesbians compared with 44 percent of gay persons).

CHOSEN FAMILIES

In addition to their families of origin, LGBT persons have other families consisting of friends, partners, and for lesbians, often ex-lovers (e.g., Dorfman et al., 1995; Kehoe, 1989; Kimmel & Sang, 1995; Raphael & Robinson, 1980; Reid, 1995; Sharp, 1997; Tully, 1988). These alternative families have been referred to as families of choice, or created families (Weinstock, 2000; Weston, 1991). Many midlife and older lesbian and gay persons were rejected by their families of origin. Even if not, they usually receive more support from their alternative families. Four-fifths (81 percent) of the midlife lesbians in

Fertitta's (1984) sample were likely to receive more support from friends, ex-lovers, and lovers than from families of origin. They were likely to retain a close link with ex-lovers much more than did heterosexual women (50 versus 25 percent). An exception is that racial and ethnic group members may not place as much value on the social support of persons outside their biological families, unless rejected by them (D'Augelli & Garnets, 1995).

In a study of the support networks of older LGB persons, Grossman et al. (2001), found that the networks averaged 6.3 persons. Close friends were the most frequently reported category, listed by 90 percent of the participants. The second most frequently reported category was partners (listed by 44 percent), followed by other relatives (39 percent), siblings (33 percent), and social acquaintances (32 percent). Co-workers were listed only by 15 percent of the participants, parents by 4 percent, and husbands/wives by 3 percent. Half (49 percent) of the members in the networks were under sixty years of age and half were sixty years of age or older; the age range was fifteen to ninety-four (average age, fifty-eight). Respondents, both male and female, were significantly older than their network members, on average by about ten years.

Of the lesbians living in Maine interviewed by Butler and Hope (1999), thirteen were in partnerships ranging in length from two to thirty-six years (mean seventeen years). Those who were partnered looked to their partners for primary support. The lesbian community was significant in the lives of about two-thirds of the sample. Pets, ex-partners, children, and birth families all contributed in varying degrees to the fabric of family. Almost all emphasized the desire for a community of friends with whom they could go through the aging process.

FRIENDS

Lesbian and gay persons who do not disclose their sexual orientation to family members or do and receive continuing negative reactions usually replace or supplement the family ties with friendship networks (Almvig, 1982; Bell & Weinberg, 1978; Francher & Henkin, 1973; Friend, 1980; Raphael & Robinson, 1980, 1981). Gay persons have significantly more close friends than heterosexual men of a similar age (Bell & Weinberg, 1978; Francher & Henkin, 1973;

Friend, 1980; Saghir & Robbins, 1973). In a study of friendships among white, middle-class lesbians at midlife, Weinstock (2000) found that friendships might have been the only family some of them could form and sustain. Friends substituted for or replaced families of origin and families with marital partners and children. Friends function as families in the day-to-day lives of these women. Among midlife lesbians with partners, friends may substitute as extended family members. Their partners are considered primary or immediate family, but they also wish to sustain close friendships. More than two-thirds (68 percent) of the older lesbian and gay persons studied by Herdt et al. (1997) had a family of choice which included a circle of close friends with whom they socialized on holidays (72 percent of the men and 63 percent of the women). Friendship networks also exist in rural areas and small towns. Fullmer, Shenk, and Eastland (1999) found, however, in a study of lesbians, that because of the paucity of lesbians in these areas, their friendship networks may include heterosexual neighbors.

Friends are more often of the same gender and ethnicity. Most of the close friends of the midlife lesbians studied by Bradford and Ryan (1991) were lesbians (64 percent) and of the same ethnicity (58 percent). Members of one's "family" studied by L. B. Brown et al. (1997) were usually of the same gender with 67 percent of older lesbians and 47 percent of older gay persons reporting that most of their friends were of the same gender. Many older lesbians studied by T. C. Jones, Nystrom, Fredriksen, Clunis, and Freeman (1999) associated primarily with other lesbians, some to the exclusion of men whether gay or heterosexual. The network of close friends studied by Quam and Whitford (1992) as mixed in gender for 65 percent of the older gay persons and 38.5 percent for the older lesbians.

In the study by Grossman et al. (2001) of LGB persons over the age of sixty, women listed significantly more persons in their networks than did men, and had more women (75 percent) in their networks (both lesbian and heterosexual) than did men (26 percent). Men's networks contained more gay/bisexual males (54 percent) than women's networks (10 percent). Heterosexual men were equally represented in men's and women's networks. Bisexual women and men reported having significantly more heterosexual persons in their networks compared to lesbian and gay respondents. An average of six people in the networks knew the participant's sexual orientation, and an average of 2.5 persons did not know or suspect it. In general, persons who knew the respondents' sexual orientation provided more satisfying support, but participants were no more satisfied with the support from others with the same sexual orientation versus those with a different sexual orientation.

When asked about the sexual orientation of their friends, in the study by Quam and Whitford (1992), more than half of the older lesbians reported that most of their closest friends were lesbians. Only 27.5 percent of the older gay persons reported that most of their friends were gay. Raphael and Robinson (1980) interviewed twenty older lesbians aged fifty and older. Half of the sample (50 percent) had close, longtime heterosexual friends but wanted to meet and be with lesbians. The older lesbian and gay persons in Berger's (1984) study divided their friends into two sets: one heterosexual, the other lesbian and gay. L. B. Brown et al. (1997) reported that their sample of older gay persons had an equal number of gay and heterosexual friends although they spent most of their time with gay friends. Herdt et al. (1997) also found that at least half of the close friends of 91 percent of their sample of older lesbian and gay persons were also lesbian or gay.

Older gay persons preferred friends of similar age. Not only did the older gay persons studied by L. B. Brown et al. (1997) spend most of their time with gay friends, but the friends were of the same age. Berger (1996) found 80 percent of gay men in his study spent half or more of leisure time with friends within ten years of their age or older. More than half had few or no friends twenty or more years younger. Most gay participants studied by L. B. Brown et al. (2001) reported that they spent 50 percent of the time or more with gay friends within their own age cohort, and their social support systems were also primarily gay persons. Lesbian friends around the same age are one of the most significant sources of support for midlife and older lesbians (Bradford & Ryan, 1991; Fertitta, 1984; Sang, 1991). Raphael and Robinson (1980) found that older lesbians sought other women of the same age for friends. Tully (1988) found in a sample of mostly white, professional, midlife lesbians a high involvement with friendship networks. Their women friends, along with partners, were the first ones they turned to for emotional support, companionship, and caregiving. Mostly this involved lesbians of their own age. D. C. Kimmel and Sang (1995) noted that both single midlife women and those with partners tended to spend social time with and receive support from other lesbians their own age. This included lovers, ex-lovers, and friends.

Benefits of Friendships

Usually, friends are the major source of social support for midlife and older lesbian and gay persons (Kurdek & Schmitt, 1987; Friend, 1987). They generally provide more social support than family-of-origin members, work colleagues, or partners (Dorfman et al., 1995; Kurdek, 1988a). Midlife lesbians who are not open with their family of origin feel closest to and most comfortable with their lesbian friends (Bradford & Ryan, 1991). Although the older lesbian and gay persons studied by Minnigerode and Adelman (1978) kept in touch with their families, they were closer to their friends. Of the forty-three gay persons in Friend's (1980) sample, many anticipated loss of family supports upon disclosure, but this did not occur. They had a broad network of both family-of-origin members and friends. Yet, their closest emotional support came from friends. The older lesbian and gay persons studied by Herdt et al. (1997) were closer to their friends than their families of origin and relied on friendship networks for support (Friend, 1980; Minnigerode & Adelman, 1978).

Friendships are also associated with various other benefits for midlife and older lesbian and gay persons. For example, they are an important source of well-being and help the adjustment process in growing older (Friend, 1980). Support from friends is associated significantly with psychological adjustment, functioning, and quality of life, not just for individual lesbian and gay persons but also for lesbian and gay couples (Kurdek, 1988b; Oetjen & Rothblum, 2000).

More than two-thirds (38 percent) of the midlife lebians studied by Sang (1991) reported that they derived both meaning and satisfaction from their friendships: 47 percent from intimate relationships, and 12 percent from children. Friendships are important in lesbians' feeling positive about themselves (e.g., D'Augelli, Collins & Hart, 1987; Weinstock, 2000). The stronger the friendship the higher the self-esteem (Raphael & Robinson, 1980, 1984).

High life satisfaction for older lesbian and gay persons is positively associated with lesbian, gay, and heterosexual friends (Adelman, 1991; J. A. Lee, 1987). They are most satisfied with the support provided by their lovers/partners and highly satisfied with the support from close friends or co-workers (Grossman et al., 2000). The older lesbian and gay participants studied by Grossman felt less lonely because of the support. Types of support received included emotional (62 percent), practical (54 percent), financial (13 percent), advice and guidance (41 percent), and general social support (72 percent). Other studies reported that high levels of companionship and mutual support were received by older lesbian and gay persons from other lesbian and gay persons (McWhirter & Mattison, 1984; Vacha, 1985). An additional benefit from this support was a diminished fear of aging (Quam & Whitford, 1992).

How Many Friends?

Most (89 percent) of the older lesbian and gay persons studied by Beeler et al. (1999) indicated that if they had a serious difficulty they could turn to at least three friends for advice and emotional support; 60 percent had six or more such friends. Friend's (1980) study of forty-three gay persons (mostly over age forty) showed that most of them (89 percent) had three close friends and that many had high-quality friendships. Only half of Bradford and Ryan's (1991) sample of midlife lesbians reported as many as five persons in their community they could talk to about personal problems. Only one such confidant was available to 8 percent of the sample. In terms of persons one could call on for a ride, 41 percent could think of as many as five, 11 percent could think of only one or none.

COUPLES

Aside from linking with friends and family, midlife and older LGB persons also want a partner and a sexual life. Most of them anticipate growing old with a partner (e.g., Bell & Weinberg, 1978; Blumstein & Schwartz, 1983; Bryant & Demian, 1994; Kurdek, 1995; Peplau, 1993; Saghir & Robbins, 1973; Tully, 1988). This primary partner is usually the central focus of one's chosen family (James & Murphy, 1998). Yet lesbian and gay couple arrangements are diverse. For example, some partners commit to each other but do not live together. Both options can be characterized by enduring bonds of intimacy and loyalty. Some partners have more than one significant partner; and some partners coexist with heterosexual marriages. Some lesbian and gay persons not currently in a relationship may be between relationships. Some may be searching for a partner but have not yet found one. Some may choose to be single for shorter or longer periods of times. Some who have only casual relationships with several others may not identify as single (Hostetler & Cohler, 1997; Hostetler, 2000; James & Murphy, 1998). Asking LGB persons to define their situations is the best way to understand the nature and personal significance of their various relationships (Cabaj & Klinger, 1996; Hostetler & Cohler, 1997).

It is also necessary to understand several factors that may affect any particular couple. This may include developmental issues such as disclosures, living and economic situations, distribution of power and resources, sexual and emotional stability, presence or absence of children, and duration of the relationship. In addition, individuals within a couple may be at various points in the life course, and they will be different from each other in terms of relationship history, degree of importance attached to relational status, access to social support, responsibility for raising children, and other factors. There are also differences in partner demographics including race/ethnicity, social class, income, and age (Hostetler, 2000).

Another source of diversity lies in what lesbian and gay couples label themselves, which could include friend, significant other, partner, lover, boyfriend, or girlfriend (Hostetler, 2000). In a national survey of mostly white lesbian (560) and gay (706) couples together an average of six years, the terms *lover* and *partner* or *life partner* were most often used. More men (40 percent) than women (30 percent) preferred the term *lover;* more women (37 percent) than men (27 percent) preferred the terms *partner* or *life partner* (Bryant & Demian, 1994). All these terms, however, may be rejected for reasons such as *partner* implying a business association and *lover* implying a main interest in sex with the other person (Berger, 1990; Murphy, 1994). Some couple members refer to themselves as *husband* or *wife*. These words suggest a more serious relationship than *friend, lover,* or *partner* (A. Martin, 1982). Yet outsiders may use a less serious word like *lover* to diminish the seriousness of lesbian and gay relationships (A. Martin, 1982). Older cohorts of lesbians may not apply any of these words to their relationships even if long-term or even call themselves lesbian (Fullmer et al., 1999). Many old-old lesbian and gay persons have never identified themselves with any of the nonhetero-sexual terms. If they had partners they referred to themselves as roommates (L. M. Woolf, 2002). Here again, it is best to ask the members of each individual couple what they prefer to call themselves (Berger, 1990). Whatever terms couples use, they may have profound meanings to the couples as well as reflect historical changes (Nardi, 1999).

Couple Models

The dominant model for couples of all cultures is of a heterosexual couple (Blumstein & Schwartz, 1983; McWhirter & Mattison, 1984). A prevalent belief is that partners in same sex-gender couples emulate these models. Thereby, they adopt the traditional heterosexual roles of either husband or wife, or one plays a masculine-dominant role and the other a feminine-submissive role (Peplau, 1982-1983; Weitz, 1989). This was the predominant couple pattern for same-sex couples in the United States from the 1920s to the early 1960s known as butch-femme (Davis & Kennedy, 1986; Faderman, 1992; Laird, 2000). It was especially common among lesbian couples during the 1950s (Nestle, 1992). In their study of working-class lesbians between the mid-1930s and early 1960s in Buffalo, New York, Kennedy and Davis (1993) found that butch-femme roles were primarily enacted through appearance and sexual expression. Butches displayed a masculine appearance in clothes and haircuts and were the doers and the givers, whereas femmes displayed feminine or even glamorous appearances and were the receivers.

Generally, the butch-femme roles of prior periods have not endured (Weston, 1996). Starting in the 1970s, lesbians could not imagine taking on these roles. The feminist and lesbian feminist movements also rejected these roles as they reflected the patriarchal system (Kennedy & Davis, 1993). This is not to say that no one in lesbian and gay communities plays traditional roles. Some persons may feel comfortable with these roles and may play out some version of them (Weber, 1996).

Another traditional model, mentor-apprentice, is still followed among a small minority of gay men. The partners are usually separated in age by five to ten years and have an arrangement whereby the older partner is the mentor or leader and makes the important decisions (Harry, 1982, 1984). Lesbians do not generally follow this pattern.

The most prevalent couple pattern today is best friends (Peplau, 1983a, 1983b), a pattern that reflects the general social shift to more flexible and egalitarian roles for couple partners (Faderman, 1991). Equality, sharing, reciprocity, companionship, and role flexibility are assumed (Kurdek & Schmitt, 1986a; J. M. Lynch & Reilly, 1986). Many lesbian and gay couples are innovative in developing rules, expectations, and divisions of labor (Peplau & Cochran, 1990). Innovations, however, can also cause stress and conflict (D. J. Patterson & Schwartz, 1994).

Relationships among bisexual persons are even more complex as they often seek several different relationship arrangements to meet sexual, romantic, and emotional needs. These arrangements can include a partner who meets many needs but is not solely responsible for all needs; different partners, each of whom meets a particular need; partners who are friends and sexual partners, but not romantic partners; and acquaintances and strangers who provide purely sexual encounters (Rust, 1996a). The most frequent ideal arrangement involves two core relationships, one heterosexual and one same sex-gender. Variations of this arrangement, from most prevalent to least prevalent, include an open link with no boundaries regarding other possible sexual partners; a primary heterosexual link (often a marriage) and secondary same sex-gender linkups; or a primary same sex-gender link and one or more secondary heterosexual links (M. S. Weinberg et al., 1994). Women prefer a person of each sex-gender to meet different emotional needs (Nichols, 1988), whereas men prefer each sex-gender primarily to meet sexual needs (Matteson, 1987). As these are ideal arrangements, many bisexual persons may never experience them (M. S. Weinberg et al., 1994).

Desire to Be Committed

A high percentage of lesbian (92 percent) and gay (96 percent) persons in couples studied by Bryant and Demian (1994) wanted to be together for life or for "a long time." Close to one-half of lesbian (48 percent) and more gay (80 percent) persons studied by Rust (1996b) indicated that they wanted a lifetime monogamous link with one partner; 30 percent of bisexual women and 15 percent of bisexual men expressed this desire.

Midlife and older lesbian and gay persons may be more serious about a committed lifelong relationship than younger persons. A sample of thirty-eight lesbians ages twenty-two to sixty-three (mean age 35.9) was studied by Rose and Zand (2000). The sample was predominantly white (8 percent African American) and middle class. The mean educational level was seventeen years. Most of the women (89 percent) were currently involved in a committed relationship with another woman. Due to age and experience, this sample of mostly midlife lesbians had different values and expectations of relationships at this mature stage in their lives. They were more purposive in attitudes and behaviors compared to when in their youth. Then, they were more casual about relationships or motivated by physical attraction, sexual gratification, or other needs unrelated to what they considered now to be important. They were now more concerned about the attachment-worthiness of a prospective partner or whether there was the necessary warmth, respect, and reciprocal liking necessary to sustain a relationship. Once they judged these attributes were present and that development of the relationship was a strong possibility, they proceeded rapidly (54 percent) and asked for a date. Many of them favored the term *courtship* over *dating* to signify that their goal was to establish a long-term relationship. The downside is that midlife lesbians may have fewer potential partners to pursue. This may cause them to escalate the course of the relationship without being sure of the compatibility of the partner. On the other hand, some midlife lesbians have doubts that a relationship will last forever because of prior experiences (M. Hall & Gregory, 1991).

MIDLIFE AND OLDER LESBIAN AND GAY COUPLES

Information on midlife and older couples is sparse. This is especially true for couples with older lesbian and gay members; much of the data come from studies done several decades ago.

Midlife Lesbians

Most lesbians tend to prefer a long-term committed relationship with one other person. There are various states of relationships ranging from seeing no one, to one woman, several women, or many women. Some couples have just met whereas others have lived together a long time and share a home and may share a family (Coss, 1991; Mitchell, 2000). Some studies found proportions of single midlife lesbians at 40 percent (Fertitta, 1984) and 33 percent (Sang, 1991). Close to three-quarters (74 percent) of the midlife lesbians studied by Bradford and Ryan (1991) were either involved in a primary linkup or dating someone. Few (19 percent) in this sample described themselves as single and uninvolved, and some gave up trying to attain partners after several attempts. Only half of the sample was living with partners, compared to 69 percent of the general population of women. As noted earlier, however, living alone does not mean one is without a partner. In interviews with eight lesbian women aged twenty-four to sixty-one, Coss (1991) reported reasons for living alone as not wanting to live openly as part of a lesbian couple or not wanting to disrupt an already satisfying life.

Sexuality

The discussion of sexuality at midlife for women is usually in the context of the menopausal transition. Yet this life transition results in few psychological or physical changes or sexual difficulties for most women whether heterosexual or lesbian. Also, the physiological changes accompanying menopause do not directly affect sexual capacity or interest (S. Hunter, Sundel, & Sundel, 2002).

A rare empirical study describing the effects of menopause on sexuality and midlife lesbians was done by E. Cole and Rothblum (1990, 1991) on a nonclinical sample of forty-one white respondents. Their ages ranged from forty-three to sixty-eight. Only 22 percent of the sample indicated that they experienced no positive changes since menopause. More than a quarter (29 percent) reported a decrease in the quality of sex. Close to half (46 percent) of the respondents, however, reported no change in the frequency of sexual activity, and the majority (76 percent) reported no sexual difficulties. More than half (56 percent) indicated no change in the frequency of orgasms. For 20 percent, orgasms were less frequent and for 22 percent they were more frequent. Changes such as taking longer to reach orgasm were not viewed as problematic.

About three-quarters of the lesbian respondents studied by E. Cole and Rothblum (1991) described their sex lives as "good" or "better than ever." Sexual activity was enjoyable, pleasurable, and satisfying. Half (50 percent) of Sang's (1993) sample of seventy-five midlife lesbians also indicated their sex lives were better than before. It was more open and exciting because of better communication and more emphasis on intimate behaviors such as touching instead of the pressure to reach orgasm.

Mildife Gay Persons

Gay persons under age fifty were found by L. B. Brown et al. (1997) to more likely be in a current or previous relationship than respondents age fifty and older. Nearly half of those midlife and older, however, involved themselves in committed relationships. These persons also felt uniformly positive about their relationships, as they provided much of the support and satisfaction in their lives.

Sexuality

When in midlife, gay persons are likely to be more sexually active than lesbians or heterosexual men and women of the same age (Kimmel & Sang, 1995). M. Pope and Schulz (1990) found that most (91 percent) of the eighty-seven gay persons they studied, ages forty to seventy, were sexually active, and that most experienced no change in sexual enjoyment compared with their earlier years (69 percent). Some (13 percent) reported increased sexual enjoyment. An earlier study by M. S. Weinberg and Williams (1974) found that gay persons aged forty-five and older reported less sexual activity than younger respondents. Gray and Dressel (1985), however, found no significant differences across age groups in the number of partners or amount of sexual activity. Blumstein and Schwartz (1983) reported that a decrease in sexual activity for both lesbian and gay persons in couples was associated more with length of the relationship than with age alone.

Bisexual Midlife Persons

In a rare study of midlife bisexual persons, M. S. Weinberg, Williams, and Pryor (2001) found that in midlife, sexual involvement decreased for these persons. Partly, this change was attributed to menopause, aging, a perceived decrease in sexual attractiveness, and distractions of other responsibilities. A move toward sexual activity with one sex-gender increased for half of the group. This was often related to the desire for monogamy.

Midlife Parenting

Few studies focus on parenting among midlife and older lesbian and gay persons. An exception was a small sample of nine midlife lesbian parents studied by C. Donaldson (2000). The partners were not interviewed. Ages of the sample ranged from forty-five to sixty-two, with a mean age of 50.7. Six were Caucasian, two African American, and one Hispanic. They were predominantly professionals and middle class. Most (six) had a professional degree. Two identified as working class. All had been in the same relationship for five to sixteen years with a mean length of eleven years. Eight were nonbiological mothers, six participants' partners carried their child, and two participants adopted children. Three had children previously, one as a single woman, one as a married woman, and one in a committed lesbian relationship. One woman gave birth at age forty-three. The age range of the children (twelve) was six weeks to eight years old with a mean age of 36.5 months.

All the midlife lesbian mothers studied by C. Donaldson (2000) reported positive feelings about their parenting experience. They all felt competent as mothers and bonded to their children. Most felt they had a level of patience and confidence in midlife that enhanced their parenting. Mostly they were satisfied with negotiated financial arrangements, child care schedules, and division of labor. They also reported a lessening of romantic and sexual intimacy between themselves and their partners following the birth or adoption of a child. Older lesbian parents (mean age 50.7) were compared with younger lesbian parents (mean age thirty-six). Both groups focused on the child more than on their partners but no one expressed concern about this. Intimacy between partners increased after the children entered school and with each passing year.

Seven of the midlife lesbian mothers from the C. Donaldson (2000) study reported greater contact with the mainstream community since having children, and five reported they were more comfortable straddling the fence between the lesbian community and the dominant mainstream community than they were when younger. Although some of the mothers experienced discrimination, most were surprised at the acceptance in the larger community. Seven described overwhelming support from their extended family of friends and from their biological families. However, all of them lived in the San Francisco Bay Area and San Jose, where residents pride themselves on acceptance and services for lesbian and gay persons.

These mothers expressed fears about economic security and their children's growing economic needs. Five women had concerns about elderly parents. Each of them felt a dual responsibility to care both for their child or children and their parents. Five expressed the fear of being unable to participate in their children's continuing development and that they would not be in good health when their children graduated, married, or had children of their own (C. Donaldson, 2000).

Older Lesbian and Gay Persons

From a 1996 study of 160 older predominantly white lesbian and gay persons in Chicago, Herdt et al. (1997) reported that 56 percent of the total sample were with a lover or partner. A greater number of lesbians (79 percent) were partnered than were gay persons (46 percent). Almost half (47 percent) of the older gay persons and 50 percent of the older lesbians studied by Grossman et al. (2001) stated that they had a current partner, and 29 percent lived with their partners. Some lived with others such as friends (2 percent) and relatives (2 percent); 3 percent said they were homeless. The coupled partners averaged 15.25 years together.

A 1999 study was conducted for SAGE consisting of 253 older lesbian and gay persons in New York City. The sample was 80 percent male, mostly white (2 percent black, 2 percent Hispanic), and the median income was $39,900. More than two-thirds (65 percent) of the sample lived alone. This was nearly twice the rate of all persons sixty-five years or older in New York City (36 percent). Fewer than one in five was currently living with a life partner in contrast to nearly half of the general older population who were currently married. Most (90 percent) of the sample had no children, versus only 20 percent of all seniors (Cross, 1999).

Close to half (48 percent) of another sample of older lesbian and gay persons lived alone, 38 percent with a partner, and 5 percent with a nonromantic roommate (Beeler et al., 1999). In other studies, somewhere between 40 and 60 percent of older gay persons and about 50 percent of older lesbians were reported to live alone (Almvig, 1982; Berger, 1996; Friend, 1980; Kehoe, 1986; Kimmel, 1979-1980; G. Weinberg, 1970). In a study of gay persons in Australia, more than half of those over age fifty lived alone—a greater proportion than in the younger age groups (Ven, Rodden, Crawford, & Kippax, 1997).

Older Lesbians

Approximately half or more of older lesbians were found in several studies not to be in a primary same sex-gender link (e.g., Almvig, 1982; Berger, 1996; Kehoe, 1986; J. Kelly, 1975; Kimmel, 1979-80; Raphael & Robinson, 1984; Silberman & Walton, 1986). According to several studies, only 18 percent of older lesbians were in a current committed link with another woman (Kehoe, 1989; Schreurs & Buunk, 1996). T. C. Jones and Nystrom (2002) found in their more recent sample of sixty-two older lesbians, that most (65 percent) had partners at the time of the interviews, while the others indicated that they were single or that their partners were deceased. Half (50 percent) had been in heterosexual marriages; 42 percent reported they had children. For those who were single, just as for midlife lesbians, the pool of potential partners may not be large.

Sexuality

Most in Deevey's (1990) sample of older lesbians reported they were still sexually active. In Bell and Weinberg's (1978) earlier study, most older lesbians were found to participate in sex although they were less sexually active than younger lesbians. For those who experienced sex with a partner, Raphael and Robinson (1980) found that older lesbians desired a strong emotional bond prior to sex. Several authors (Adelman, 1980; Kehoe, 1986; Raphael & Robinson, 1980; Tully, 1983) noted that at times women had a strong emotional bond between each other and no sex. Loulan (1987) found, however, that lesbians over age sixty experienced sex with their partners two to five times a month, more than any other age group in the study.

Most studies reported that although sex was important to older lesbians it may not be of utmost importance (e.g., Kehoe, 1986, 1989; Raphael & Robinson, 1984). Kehoe (1989) asked lesbians in her sample how important sex was to them in a relationship before and after age sixty. Prior to sixty, only one person indicated that it was the major part. It was one of other important parts for 84 percent, unimportant to 13 percent. Two women were celibate. After age sixty, 72 percent rated sex as one important part of their relationships and 28 percent unimportant. No one considered sex as the main part of a relationship. The importance of friendship and intimacy surpassed the importance of sex for most of the respondents. After age seventy, it was not easy for lesbians to find sexual partners. The desire was still there, however, and seeking sexual partners continued (Raphael & Robinson, 1980).

Older Gay Men

In several studies, approximately 70 percent of older gay men were found not to be in a primary same sex-gender link (e.g., Berger, 1996; J. Kelly, 1975; Kimmel, 1979-1980; Silberman & Walton, 1986). Berger (1982/1996) found that two-fifths of older gay persons lived with a partner, about one-third currently were in an exclusive sexual relationship with another man, and more than half had an exclusive sexual relationship at some time in the past. Older gay persons were less likely to live with a partner/spouse, and less likely to be exclusive with their sexual partner compared to heterosexual men. Several other early studies reported progressive declines in primary partnerships as gay persons aged (e.g., Kimmel, 1978). One study reported that the primary relationships of gay persons reached their greatest numbers between ages forty-five to fifty-five and declined after that to close to none (J. Kelly, 1975). A more recent study reported that 24 percent of older gay persons were in same sex-gender relationships (Quam & Whitford 1992). Most older gay American Indians reported being in or having been in long-term same sex-gender relationships (L. B. Brown et al., 2001).

Sexuality

Older gay men reported lower levels of sexual activity and interest than midlife men (M. Pope & Schulz, 1990). Sexual interest does not decrease with age for gay men but older gay men experience a decrease in frequency of sexual outlets and frequency of sex as they age (e.g., Bell & Weinberg, 1978; Kimmel, 1979; J. A. Lee, 1990). More than two-thirds of a sample of older gay persons reported on by L. B. Brown et al. (1997) experienced fewer than two sexual encounters a month; but, in Berger's (1996) study of older gay persons, almost two-thirds (60 percent) reported experiencing sex once a week or more often. Of those who were sexually active, 57 percent were with only one partner during the six months prior to the study. Less than one-quarter of the sample had three or more partners during the prior six months.

The Impact of HIV/AIDS

Many studies on sexual activity in gay relationships were done prior to the HIV/AIDS crisis that dramatically changed the gay community. The crisis reduced the number of available mates, and instilled the need to negotiate safe sex and to decide to be monogmous. Gay men feared the possibility of being infected by their partner or infecting him, and coping with the illness and likely death of one's partner or oneself (Hostetler, 2000).

Knowledge and the kinds of attitudes and beliefs gay and bisexual men fifty to eighty years of age and older had about HIV/AIDS was studied by Kooperman (1994). The sample included 139 gay persons from the United States, Canada, and Australia, but was over-represented by men who lived in San Francisco. Two-thirds of the sample (66 percent) reported considerable concern about AIDS, 21 percent some concern. More than half (62 percent) reported that they knew between one and ten people diagnosed with AIDS. Others (19 percent) knew between eleven and twenty people living with AIDS or who died from it.

Gay persons studied by Kooperman (1994) acknowledged that their behavior had to change because of the HIV/AIDS crisis. They were knowledgeable about how HIV was transmitted and participated in low-risk sexual activity. Most (88 percent) talked to their sexual partners about the types of sexual activity they were unwilling to engage in to reduce the risk of infection. The rate of anal intercourse without a condom, generally considered one of the riskiest sexual activities for gay and bisexual men, was reduced to a low frequency. In contrast, the rate of low-risk activities was high, such as mutual masturbation.

The fear of AIDS may interfere with developing relationships. Some gay persons may avoid all sexual contact (Linde, 1994). L. S. Brown et al. (1997) reported that some gay persons did not socialize much with persons with HIV/AIDS since they were going to lose them, or if they did socialize, the disease interfered with intimacy. Most of them indicated that the quantity of their sexual activity also decreased, attributable partly to risk of HIV/AIDS. Some were now celibate. Other gay persons explored more erotic activity and less sex. The focus was also more on character and spiritual development than the purely physical aspects of these links. Yet, almost three-quarters of the sample studied by Kooperman (1994) had sexual activity during the thirty days prior to the survey.

Satisfaction and Other Benefits of Being in a Couple

When studies compare lesbian and gay couples with heterosexual couples, no discrepancies are found in quality (Kurdek, 1994, 1995), cohesion (Green, Bettinger, & Zacks, 1996), closeness (Peplau & Cochran, 1990), adjustments (Kurdek, 1995), or satisfaction (e.g., Kurdek, 1994, 1995; Peplau & Cochran, 1990). For some samples, same sex-gender relationships were more satisfiying than prior heterosexual relationships. For example, the relationships of older lesbians studied by Kehoe (1989) were more caring, gentle, emotionally close, and sexually satisfying than prior heterosexual linkups. In addition, compared to earlier same sex-gender relationships, their current same sex-gender relationships were less intense, quieter, and more stable. Schreurs and Buunk (1996) found that the older the participants were in lesbian couples, the more satisfied they were. Silverstein (1981) found in a study of gay couples that older couples were the most content.

Both J. A. Lee (1987) and Berger (1980, 1996) found that a lover or exclusive sex partner was highly related to satisfaction in old age for gay persons. Older gay persons in long-term partnerships were more likely to be satisfied with their lives than those who chose an unattached single life. Yet although Lee (1987) reported that all the men living with partners, with one exception, were among the happiest men in his sample, twenty-six other happy men were not in couples.

Lee also noted that an enduring linkup did not necessarily have to be with a lover or even with someone who was lesbian or gay. There can be different arrangements that are also happy. Bell and Weinberg (1978) reported, for example, that the happiest men in their sample were in a close-coupled link (little outside sexual activity) but that those in another type of couple arrangement, functional, were almost as happy (95 versus 99 percent). Participants in the functional type of couple were not in a partnership with each other but experienced sex several or more times a week.

Most older gay persons in other studies rated their current sex lives as satisfactory (Berger, 1984, 1992, 1996; J. Kelly, 1977; Kimmel, 1978). Half of Kimmel's respondents felt that sex was more satisfactory older than when younger. In a sample of gay persons ages forty to seventy-seven, M. L. Pope and Schulz (1990) found that most older respondents reported levels of sexual satisfaction remaining high since young adulthood. Berger (1992) reported that most older gay persons talked about sex as qualitatively different, with less focus on the sexual act. Although the pace of sexual activity may slow down in later years, satisfaction may be greater. In Lee's (1987) sample, the happier men were satisfied with their sex lives.

Some studies have reported positive benefits beyond general satisfaction for older gay participants in couples. Berger (1980, 1996) found that having and maintaining a satisfactory close relationship was among the variables that related to adjustment for older gay persons. Grossman et al. (2000) reported that older LGB persons who lived with a partner reported less loneliness and better physical and emotional health (e.g., Kimmel, 1977). L. B. Brown et al. (1997) reported that having a partner in a monogamous relationship was associated not only with life satisfaction but higher levels of psychosocial adaptation and self-esteem for older gay persons.

DURATION OF LINKS

Comparative studies of heterosexual marriages and lesbian and gay partnerships reveal few differences in duration or factors leading to dissolution (Hostetler, 2000). Almost half (47 percent) of heterosexual marriages end by the fifth anniversary (Bumpass & Sweet, 1989). The average length of time together for the sample of lesbian and gay couples studied by Haas and Stafford (1998) was five and one-half years. Yet several studies found lesbian and gay couples who had been together ten years or longer (e.g., Bryant & Demian, 1994; B. Johnson, 1990; McWhirter & Mattison, 1984). In anecdotal accounts, older lesbian and gay persons reported that relationships lasting twenty to thirty years or longer were common (e.g., Adelman, 1986; Clunis & Green, 2000; Kehoe, 1989; McWhirter & Mattison; 1984; Silverstein, 1981). Older gay persons had fewer sexual partners and a lower frequency of sex, but longer links than younger gay persons (Bell & Weinberg, 1978; Berger, 1996; Harry & DeVall, 1978; Kimmel, 1978; Saghir & Robbins, 1973; Silverstein, 1981; M. S. Weinberg & Williams, 1974). Peplau and Amaro (1982) reported that this pattern of establishing relatively stable, enduring relationships characterized most lesbian relationships as well. Longevity in itself might lead to continued longevity (Kehoe, 1989). Breakups are rare in couples together for more than ten years (Blumstein & Schwartz, 1983). Without marriage and divorce records for lesbian and gay couples, however, longevity of relationships is not fully known (Peplau, 1993).

For couples who do not last, exchange theory attempts to explain what happens on the way to broken commitments. Commitment can rise or fall depending on two factors: (1) positive attractions associated with the partner and the relationship, such as love or satisfaction, or decline in these attractions, and (2) barriers that make termination costly, such as investments in the relationship or financial costs of termination or low barriers (Levinger, 1982). Lesbian and gay couples and married heterosexual couples generally do not differ in levels of positive attractions. Married heterosexual partners, however, have stronger barriers to leaving their relationship than either gay or lesbian partners, including joint investments, the cost of divorce, possible negative effects on children, and less earning power of wives (Kurdek & Schmitt, 1986b).

Every couple is vulnerable to broken commitments because of the decline in positive attractions. Two categories of internal factors can play a role in this decline for any couple. Examples include lack of communication or support, desire to be independent, unrealistic expectations, and unfulfilled expectations. Examples of possible interpersonal factors include mismatches between partners, not having the same interests, and not talking things out. Hunter and Hickerson (2003) identified a number of other factors in these two categories.

A wider social context also affects the formation and maintenance of coupled relationships (Kitzinger & Coyle, 1995). Certain external factors may negatively affect any couple, such as the intrusion of work responsibilities, but lesbians and gay couples also face distinct challenges to their relationships because of their sexual orientation. Although external to couples, these challenges can create internal difficulties that interfere with or destroy happiness. These include cultural heterosexism that condemns same sex-gender partnerships and sexuality (Kitzinger & Coyle, 1995); few role models of successful relationships (Blando, 2001); lack of binding social arrangements that come with legal marriage (Rutter & Schwartz, 2000); and lack of support from families and friends (Bryant & Demian, 1994). These external obstacles can create negative effects for lesbian and gay couples such as internalization of negative beliefs and images of hiding and passing (Hunter & Hickerson, 2003).

The Severing of Couples

No different from other persons, lesbian and gay persons begin linkups with high hopes for a lifetime of love and closeness but often end up with dissolved linkups. If family and heterosexual friends know about the breakup of a lesbian or gay couple, they may not show support and sympathy (Becker, 1988). Lesbian and gay persons who are closeted and grieving lost relationships may disclose their sexual orientation for the first time so that they can get support from others in their community (Browning, Reynolds, & Dwonkin 1991). If they remain hidden, they grieve the loss by themselves (Becker, 1988).

SUMMARY

Few studies have been done on midlife and older lesbian and gay persons and their families of origin. There is often a mix of harmony and friction but many families become more accepting of their lesbian or gay child over time. By midlife or older age, there may be more contact. Lesbian and gay family members may play special roles in their family of origin such as caregiver of an older parent, but the literature is minimal on this topic. Chosen families made up of friends, partners, and often for lesbians, ex-lovers, are usually more important to lesbian and gay persons, especially if they were rejected by their family of origin. The benefits of friends are many, such as better quality of life and life satisfaction. Most lesbian and gay persons also want a partner. Not much is known about midlife and older couples or the literature is dated; even less is known about midlife and older lesbian and gay persons who are parenting children. The research that exists shows that being in a couple has major benefits such as increased life satisfaction, less loneliness, better physical and mental health, and higher self-esteem. Similar to heterosexual couples, not all lesbian and gay couples last. The reasons for this are similar to those among heterosexual couples except for the impact of heterosexism on lesbian and gay couples. Probably the saddest ending is when a grieving partner is not "out" and is grieving the loss by oneself.

PART III:
POSITIVES VERSUS DOWNTURNS

Chapter 5

Positives

Stereotypes about lesbian and gay persons include that they will end up in old age alone, lonely, unhappy, and depressed. Much of the research centers on countering these negative stereotypes. Though variation exists, many studies have shown that most older lesbian and gay participants do not match the negative stereotypes attributed to them (e.g., Dawson, 1982; Dorfman et al., 1995; Francher & Henkin, 1973; Friend, 1980; Kehoe, 1986; J. Kelly, 1977; Kimmel, 1977, 1978; L. B. Brown et al., 1996).

POSITIVES FOR OLDER LESBIAN AND GAY PERSONS

Adjustment and Life Satisfaction

A model developed by Friend (1990, 1991), focuses on varying routes of identity development displayed by older lesbian and gay persons. Although the historical period in which they grew up was hostile and oppressive, *affirmative* older lesbian and gay persons constructed a positive identity. They did this by refusing to accept the heterosexist ideology of the larger culture and constructing an identity on their own terms as positive, valuable, and having advantages for them (Friend, 1991). Most of these persons also reported that they were close to their families and in frequent communication with them. They were likely open with their families about their sexual identities and accepted by them. Family members were encouraged to challenge heterosexism through participation in groups such as PFLAG (Friend, 1990).

Other older lesbian and gay persons did not attain a positive identity. Some capitulated to the negative beliefs and attitudes about their sexual identities and incorporated them into beliefs and feelings about themselves. These *conforming* older lesbian and gay persons matched the negative stereotypes of older lesbian and gay persons as alienated, lonely, and depressed. They lived with self-loathing, shame, and guilt, and hid all or parts of their sexual identities from families and friends. They created a wall of separation and distance between themselves and others, having minimal and superficial contact with them (Friend, 1991). They also maintained distance from other lesbian and gay persons and were unlikely to develop social or emotional support systems with them. They did not challenge heterosexist beliefs about themselves largely because of their separation from affirmative lesbian and gay persons (Friend, 1990). Older gay black persons who viewed their sexual attractions as a disease or sin were found by Icard (1996) to not associate with black or white gay persons. Conforming persons were also likely to perceive that their stigmatized sexual orientation caused them to fail in their careers and relationships with partners and others (Adelman, 1991).

The *passing* option makes up the middle range of Friend's (1990) model. Though members of this group were not much different from those in the conforming group, they were a little less isolated, marginally accepted their sexual identities, and did not totally accept society's negative views of themselves. Yet they could not fully accept their sexual identities, partly because they capitulated to heterosexist views. They felt valued for what others expected them to be instead of whom they really were (Minton & McDonald, 1983-1984). They were often heterosexually married and closeted, passing as heterosexual. Many kept their distance from identifiable lesbian and gay persons, although some interacted with others like themselves and sometimes participated in a long-term primary link with someone of the same sex-gender. If they were in a same sex-gender relationship, however, they still presented themselves as if heterosexual. They did this by living in two worlds, one public and one secret. The emotional costs of this incongruent life, however, were often high (Friend, 1991).

Mostly open lesbian and gay persons who are affirmative about themselves are willing to participate in research. Other older lesbian and gay persons are difficult to find as they are still mostly hidden (Friend, 1990; Quam, 1993). Little is known about this group or those who are working class, nonwhite, or live outside major metropolitan areas (Hostetler, 2000). Kehoe (1989) found that many older lesbians living in rural areas and lacking transportation feel isolated and lonely.

Older lesbian and gay persons who are affirmative attained high levels of psychological adjustment (e.g., Adelman, 1991; Almvig, 1982; Berger, 1980, 1996; Dawson, 1982; Dunker, 1987; Francher & Henkin, 1973; Friend, 1980, 1987; Kehoe, 1986; J. Kelly, 1977; Kimmel, 1977, 1978; Raphael & Robinson, 1984). They seem happy, generally satisfied with their lives and adapt well to getting older (e.g., Adelman, 1988; Almvig, 1982; Berger, 1980, 1996; Deevey, 1990; Friend, 1991; T. C. Jones et al., 1999; Kehoe, 1986, 1989; Raphael & Robinson, 1984). They do not experience any significant decrease in self-acceptance as they get older nor do loneliness, anxiety, or depression increase (Berger, 1980, 1996). Most of them recognize the positive aspects of their identity and feel satisfied with themselves (J. A. Lee, 1987; Quam & Whitford, 1992).

An example of one sample in which adjustment and life satisfaction were a focus includes the thirty-nine lesbian and forty-one gay persons studied by Quam and Whitford (1992). They lived in a midwestern metropolitan area of the United States. Overall these respondents, all over age fifty, tended to score high on measures of life satisfaction, current health, and acceptance of the aging process. About half of the sample (50.65 percent) scored 75 percent or higher on life satisfaction items. The mean score was 72 percent which was close to what Berger (1980) found (74.5 percent). Forty-two percent were somewhat accepting and 35 percent very accepting of their own aging process. Three items positively associated with acceptance of the aging process were involvement in the community, participation in social organizations, and current good health.

Respondents in another sample from the Chicago Study of Lesbian and Gay Adult Development and Aging were age sixty and older (Cohler, Hostetler, & Boxer, 1998; Hostetler & Cohler, 1997; Herdt et al., 1997). They were found to be adjusting exceptionally well to later life. A majority were in long-term committed relationships. They did not report experiencing stigma related to either being gay or older. Most had lived their adult lives "below radar" or were quietly gay and not visibly involved in the institutional lesbian and gay community.

Comparison Groups

Starting in the 1970s, older lesbian and gay persons have been compared with other groups in terms of adjustment. These persons reported better self-concepts and tended to be more psychologically stable than younger lesbian and gay persons (Kehoe, 1989; Lee, 1990). Older gay persons studied by M. S. Weinberg and C. J. Williams (1974) had better self-concepts and more psychological stability than their younger counterparts. A sample of 1,100 older gay persons studied by G. Weinberg (1970) was as well adjusted as younger gay persons. The psychological adjustment of older lesbian and gay persons was also not different from that of older heterosexual persons. Minnigerode, Adelman, and Fox (1980) compared lesbian, gay, and heterosexual persons aged sixty and older. Few discrepancies were noted in psychological adjustment among the different groups. Minnigerode and Adelman (1976) also found no differences in morale among these comparison groups. Dorfman et al. (1995) reported that there were no differences among these groups in rates of depression. Generally, then, older lesbian and gay persons are as well adjusted as their heterosexual counterparts and younger lesbian and gay persons.

Contributions to Adjustment and Satisfaction

The research findings on the adjustment and satisfaction of older lesbian and gay persons identified various contributing factors. Different combinations of these factors might have allowed these persons to more easily adjust in later life and to experience satisfaction in life.

Mastery of Independence

Older lesbian and gay persons have been self-sufficient and independent much of their lives. Earlier findings (e.g., Berger, 1985; Francher & Henkin, 1973) indicated that "mastery of independence" was one of the qualities that assisted older gay persons to adjust to old age, More recent findings have confirmed this. Both older lesbian and gay persons learned to become independent, fend for themselves, and plan carefully for their older years (Berger & Kelly, 1986a, 1986b; Friend, 1991; Kimmel & Sang, 1995; Quam & Whitford, 1992; D. G.

Wolf, 1982). They also already knew how to negotiate systems needed for services (Adelman, 1991; Fassinger, 1995, 1996; Friend, 1990; Quam & Whitford, 1992).

Mastery of Stigma and Crisis Competence

Many researchers have proposed that successful resolution of the crises of coming out and disclosure, and mastering ridicule and ostracism, prepare a lesbian or gay person to cope with later life crises or to be more resilient (e.g., Berger, 1980, 1996, 1982, 1984; Berger & Kelly, 1996; Dawson, 1982; Francher & Henkin, 1973; Friend, 1987, 1990; Kehoe, 1986; Kimmel, 1978, 1979-1980, 1993; J. A. Lee, 1987; McDougall, 1993; Minnigerode et al., 1980; Sharpe, 1997; Quam & Whitford, 1992; Vacha, 1985; Weeks, 1983; M. S. Weinberg & Williams, 1974). Compared to older heterosexual persons who face devaluation for the first time because of ageism, older lesbian and gay persons have already learned to cope with devaluation because of their sexual identity (L. B. Brown et al., 2001). Some researchers, however, have raised questions about the association of crisis competence with adjustment and satisfaction.

Although some of the exceedingly satisfied gay persons, aged fifty to eighty, in J. A. Lee's (1987, 1989) study experienced long periods of identity crisis, some men who did not go through a crisis of this type were unhappy; and, the happiest participants reported the fewest numbers of crises. Self-acceptance developed more easily for them than other participants. No evidence was found by M. S. Weinberg and Williams (1974) that if gay persons combat stigma and prejudice their capacity to manage the biological aspects of aging, such as illness and infirmity will increase. Reid (1995) indicated that the coming out and disclosure processes can lead to personal growth and development, and they can also overwhelm persons and their coping resources. R. M. Berger (1996) suggested that if multiple, difficult crises were not quickly and effectively resolved; they could deplete one's social and emotional resources. Presumably the ability to cope well with subsequent stressors in life might also be jeopardized.

Theories that require the necessity of surviving suffering earlier in life so that old age can be a positive and satisfying experience were especially disparaged by J. A. Lee (1987). Although a man in Lee's study with one of the highest incomes had very low life satisfaction, generally income level was closely associated with life satisfaction. Wealthy gay persons tended to fare better because they could obtain more resources. Instead of using the old Puritan ethic to explain a good result later in life, the real "crisis competence" for older gay persons or any other persons includes "good health, social class advantage, and exchange power, often enhanced by alliance with a significant other" (p. 60). The crisis competence hypothesis also does not consider cohort effects on lesbian and gay persons. When current midlife and younger cohorts reach later life, issues related to sexual orientation may be much less significant than now (Hostetler, 2000). Nor are other factors considered, such as social support and certain personality characteristics (e.g., hardiness and self-esteem) that have been found to moderate the negative effects of stress (DiPlacido, 1998).

Sex-Gender Role Flexibility

Lesbian and gay persons potentially feel more freedom to behave in flexible ways because they are not bound to traditional sex-gender roles (Fassinger, 1997). When older, they can take care of themselves because they have performed tasks all their adult lives associated with both sex-genders such as financial management, shopping, and cooking (Friend, 1991). Learning these skills earlier in life makes life transitions (e.g., losing a partner) easier (L. B. Brown et al., 2001). Lesbians feel strengthened to cope with later life because of not following the social prescriptions for women. Many mental health difficulties experienced by women, such as depression, seem to be associated with characteristics of their sex-gender role socialization, including passiveness, dependency, and performing powerless roles (Fassinger, 1997; Sharp, 1997).

Satisfaction with Sexual Identity

Various researchers have found an association between adjustment to aging among older lesbian and gay persons and satisfaction with their sexual identity (Adelman, 1991; Friend, 1990; Quam, 1993). Most of the older lesbian and gay persons studied by Grossman et al. (2001) mastered sexual identity challenges leading to identity acceptance, identity pride, or identity synthesis (Cass, 1979), and have become members of social groups of older LGBT persons. Yet, positive identity was sometimes not achieved until after years of struggle with heterosexism and discrimination (Adelman, 1991; Minnigerode et al., 1980).

Respondents who attained a positive identity tended to talk about self-acceptance and the advantages of their sexual orientation. A major characteristic of respondents who reported lower satisfaction was their perception that their sexual orientation was associated with failures in their careers and relationships (both friends and partners) (Adelman, 1991). These results confirmed findings in earlier studies (G. Weinberg, 1972) that internalization of, or rejection of, negative stereotypes associated with same sex-gender sexual identity leads to being less well adjusted, or well adjusted.

In describing personal and psychological changes associated with getting older, gay participants studied by Kertzner (1999) most frequently mentioned an increase in self-acceptance. This was often linked to an acceptance of their gay identity, although sometimes it was related to an increased sense of proficiency in work or a heightened appreciation of their importance to others as friend, family member, or volunteer. Many of these men also pointed to their greater comfort with self-disclosure of their sexual identity, although several men were not sure if this reflected personal change or an increased social tolerance of gay persons. Regardless, some men in the study felt that being gay made it harder to get older. The reasons included decreased social supports, the absence of traditional family life, and the lack of children who were seen as providing a distraction from the aging process.

Sequence of Developmental Events

The sequence of developmental events was found by Adelman (1991), in a sample of twenty-five lesbians (mean age sixty-four) and twenty-seven gay persons (mean age sixty-five), to have a significant association with adjustment to aging. Experimentation with being lesbian or gay prior to self-definition was related to high life satisfaction, low self-criticism, and few psychosomatic complaints. The reverse sequence (self-definition prior to experimentation) was related to low satisfaction and high self-criticism. Experimention appears to be an adaptive pattern because it allows internal adjustment to stigma prior to self-definition (Dank, 1971; de Monteflores & Schultz,

1978), and time to develop skills to cope with stigma. If, however, future cohorts grow up in more supportive environments, this experimentation stage may not be required for adjustment (Adelman, 1991).

Disclosure or No Disclosure

After the Stonewall rebellion, lesbian and gay persons were more willing to speak out about their sexual identities. Some studies found that no disclosure, however, was associated with more favorable adjustment among older lesbian and gay persons (e.g., Adelman, 1991; Friend, 1990; J. A. Lee, 1987; Quam, 1993).

Adjustment to later life or high life satisfaction for older lesbian and gay persons was also related to low disclosure at work. Those with a low disclosure style reported that work was important while the opposite was reported for those with a high disclosure style. Those who did not disclose, however, felt that they had to work harder or achieve more because of their sexual orientation. This is not unusual conduct in stigmatized groups (Goffman, 1963). Achievement may increase the value of work which then increases the fear of discrimination and low disclosure. Compartmentalization also characterized those undisclosed at work. Personal life is never discussed at work. This reticence might also represent a cohort factor, as this generation did not discuss their personal life no matter what their sexual orientation was (Adelman, 1991).

Results from other studies contradicted the results cited previously about disclosure. Berger (1996) found emotional difficulties associated with low disclosure among older gay persons. An early study by M. S. Weinberg and Williams (1974) found older gay persons were less concerned about the exposure of their sexual orientation than were younger gay persons.

Community Participation

As discussed in Chapter 3, older gay persons who actively participate in activities in the lesbian and gay community appear to enjoy higher levels of psychological well-being (Berger, 1996; Francher & Henkin, 1973; J. A. Lee, 1987; Quam & Whitford, 1992). For example, the men in Berger's study reported higher levels of morale than are found among older persons generally (Havighurst, Neugarten, & Tobin, 1961).

Mental Health

Most research has so far not discovered higher prevalences of mental health difficulties among older LGBT persons than among heterosexual persons. One study of 108 older heterosexual and lesbian and gay persons in urban central and southern California did not find significant differences in depression or social isolation. Heterosexuals derived more support from family while older LGBT persons generally gained more support from friends (Dorfman et al., 1995). In another study, older gay persons were comparable or healthier than their heterosexual peers regarding life satisfaction, and few reported serious depression or anxiety (Berger, 1980). Dorfman also found no significant differences among lesbian, gay, and heterosexual persons in depression or loneliness. More than half of Kehoe's (1986, 1989) sample of older lesbians rated their mental health as good to excellent.

Mental health was studied by D'Augelli et al. (2001) and Grossman et al. (2001) in their samples of older lesbian and gay persons (age sixty and older). The vast majority (84 percent) of the sample said their mental health was good or excellent; 14 percent fair, 2 percent poor, and fewer than 1 percent very poor. About 12 percent reported a deterioration in mental health in the past five years, but more than one-third said it was somewhat or much better. About 10 percent reported a mental illness or disability, and 18 percent of these persons said they required medication. Both current alcohol use and drug use were low. Only 9 percent could be categorized as problem drinkers. There was no evidence of drug abuse.

Predictors of mental health were also explored by D'Augelli et al. (2001) and Grossman et al. (2001). Consistent with the findings of Berger (1996) and Kehoe (1989), the large majority of older participants reported fairly high levels of self-esteem and low levels of internalized oppression. Most (80 percent) were glad to be lesbian, gay, or bisexual while 8 percent reported being depressed about their sexual orientation. Some (17 percent) wished they were heterosexual and 9 percent had sought counseling to stop same sex-gender feelings. Participants had not often considered suicide due to their sexual orientation.

Better current mental health in the studies done by D'Augelli et al. (2001) and Grossman et al. (2001) was significantly associated with higher current income, better health, higher cognitive functioning,

higher self-esteem, more positive views of sexual orientation, less suicidal feelings because of one's sexual orientation, less loneliness, and
more control over loneliness. Self-esteem was also positively related to
income and a greater number of persons in one's support networks, but
was inversely related to experiences of victimization because of sexual
orientation. Self-rating of mental health was also inversely related to
experiences of victimization. Older LGB adults who reported living
with partners had better overall current mental health, higher self-
esteem, less suicidal thinking in the past year, and were less lonely
compared to those who lived alone. Those who were parents were also
less lonely, felt significant personal responsibility for loneliness, and
reported more positive change in their mental health in the past five
years than nonparents (Grossman et al., 2001). Less decline in mental
health over the past five years was predicted by better health and cognitive functioning and by a higher percentage of persons who knew the
participant's sexual orientation.

Participants studied by D'Augelli et al. (2001) who acknowledged a
mental disorder, rated their emotional and mental health lower and reported more lifetime suicidal ideation. Older gay persons scored significantly higher on personal discomfort with their sexual orientation
and on thinking about suicide because of sexual orientation. They also
showed more evidence of alcohol abuse and compared to 4 percent of
lesbians, 11 percent of gay persons would be considered problem drinkers. They more often felt that persons are responsible for their own
loneliness.

Cognitive Functioning

Cognitive changes in late life may be the most significant source of
personal distress. However, a majority (84 percent) of the D'Augelli
et al. (2001) sample of older lesbian and gay persons described their
abilities to think clearly and concentrate as good or excellent. Approximately 68 percent reported that their cognitive functioning had
not changed in the past five years, 30 percent that their ability to think
clearly had improved. Many (73 percent) also indicated that their
memory was good or excellent. While almost one-third (29 percent)
reported their memory had become somewhat worse in the past five
years, almost two-thirds (65 percent) reported their memory had
stayed about the same during the previous five years. Older participants reported having poorer memory than younger participants.

Physical Health

In their sample of sixty-two older lesbians, T. C. Jones and Nystrom (2002) found that the vast majority (94 percent) reported their health to be either excellent or good. Slightly over a quarter (27 percent), however, indicated that they had a major disability or health problem of some kind. Mostly, the older lesbian and gay participants in the study done by D'Augelli et al. (2001) and Grossman et al. (2001) were also in good physical health. Three-fourths (75 percent) of the participants studied by Grossman et al. (2001) reported that their physical health was good or excellent, 21 percent fair, 4 percent poor. Regarding changes in physical health status over the past five years, 11 percent said that their health was better, 50 percent that it stayed the same, and 30 percent that it became worse. Only 11 percent described their health status as interfering with life activities. More than half (57 percent) indicated that they exercised regularly, 27 percent sometimes, 12 percent seldom, and 4 percent never. There was apparently no difference in reported physical health between men and women, or between lesbian, gay, and bisexual persons. Those living with a partner reported significantly better physical health than those living alone. Age was unrelated to overall health, but was significantly, if weakly, associated with health interfering with daily activities. Physical health was also related to household income; those reporting better physical health had higher incomes. Their health also interfered less with their activities. Those experiencing less lifetime victimization reported better physical health. Physical health status was related (not signficantly) to the number of persons in one's support networks; those who had more persons in their networks reported better physical health.

POSITIVES IN MIDLIFE

Midlife Lesbians

Recent research findings on the experiences of midlife lesbians indicate that midlife can be a transformative time (Hostetler, 2000). In addition, lesbians have similarities with midlife women in the general population. Although this period of life is not without its difficulties, midlife women with economic advantages and college educations can particularly experience new and exciting opportunities, unexpected pleasures, and greater self-esteem and self-acceptance (Baruch and Brooks-Gunn, 1984). Mitchell and Helson (1990) went so far as to proclaim midlife, more specifically the middle of this period of life (the early fifties), the prime time of life for women. Women's roles are changing, and they are experiencing freed up energy (Haan, 1989). This period of life also appears to be a prime time for midlife lesbians. In Sang's (1990, 1991, 1992a, 1992b, 1993) study of 110 mostly white, middle-class, self-identified lesbians between the ages of forty and fifty-nine (average age of forty-seven), three-quarters (76 percent) felt that midlife was the best period of their lives. Three-quarters (76 percent) were more self-confident and self-directed than when they were younger. Based on effective coping with the past, they felt confidence and optimism about the future. In addition, they felt increased wisdom, power, and freedom. Earlier, Fertitta (1984) found similar positive changes at midlife in her sample of sixty-eight, white, child-free, never-married midlife lesbians. The changes included more self-acceptance and gained perspective and wisdom.

Specific themes were identified in Sang's (1991) research that corresponded with positive changes at midlife for lesbians: feeling more comfortable with themselves and more self-accepting; wanting more play and fun versus pushing so much to strive at work; more risk taking and confidence to try new things; increased self-knowledge and self-discovery; renewed dreams or a sense of renewal related to previous interests, suppressed aspects of the self, or new passions; changes, doing things differently, and refocus; spending more time on meaningful activities; more self-confidence, self-directedness, and authenticity; and balancing the various aspects of their lives.

The twenty-one lesbians studied by Butler and Hope (1999) ages fifty-four to seventy-four (mean of fifty-nine years) were mostly in good health, satisfied with health care, and felt positive about their lives. They generally did not feel old. On average, they had lived in rural Maine for eighteen years. For many, the beauty of Maine attracted them and their surroundings continued to contribute to their well-being. Many lived independent lives that they saw as authentic for them.

Midlife lesbians, as do their midlife heterosexual counterparts, risk development of chronic difficulties and possibly degenerative diseases with accompanying costly care. This includes depression (10 percent), anxiety (6 percent), alcohol (4 percent), cancer (1 percent), and other drugs (1 percent) (Bradford & Ryan, 1991). Most midlife lesbians surveyed by Bradford and Ryan, however, reported few if any complaints about physical health. Four out of five perceived their health to be excellent or good. This was different from midlife women in the general population where 88 percent rated their overall health from good to excellent. In terms of the complaints that existed, differences between the general population of midlife women and midlife lesbians, respectively, included high blood pressure (13 percent versus 9 percent), heart and/or circulatory problems (8 percent versus 5 percent), arthritis (9 percent versus 23 percent), hemorrhoids (1 percent versus 7 percent), and obesity (63 percent versus 30 percent). The two groups had the same proportion of reported diabetes (about 2 percent). Sang (1993) also found that weight gain was an issue for 16 percent of her sample of midlife lesbians. The most commonly reported health problems in the midlife lesbian sample were obesity, arthritis, back trouble, and allergies (Bradford & Ryan, 1991).

Midlife Gay Persons

A small exploratory study of thirty midlife gay person's self-appraisals of being gay was done by Kertzner (2001). These men were relatively affluent, mostly white, and well educated. The average age was 45.6. Close to half (thirteen) were in relationships with a median duration of five years; the range was from three months to nineteen years. Seven were HIV positive and three untested. Two had fathered children but had not played an active role in raising them. During midlife, they experienced high levels of commitment to their sexual identity, self-esteem, and life satisfaction. Eleven said these were the best years of their lives. The most frequent response to what was important in their lives was friendships or relationships, endorsed by twenty of the men, followed by work and personal philosophy about life. Seven mentioned being out or open. For many of the thirteen men in relationships, the meaning of a gay identity was inextricably tied to the history and current state of their partnerships. (See Kooden and Flowers [2000] for an extensive guide on how gay persons can thrive at midlife.)

Kertzner (1999) also examined the themes of coherence and reconciliation in the context of how midlife gay men evaluated their present and past life experiences. Coherence was rated by a sense of meaning in their lives, social validation of personal experience by others, and a sense of continuity between earlier and present life experiences (Cohler, 1982). Reconciliation was rated by pervasiveness of regret in self-appraisals, attitudes about past mistakes, and ability to relinquish unrealistic expectations in life appraisals (Levinson, Darrow, Klein, Levinson, & McKee, 1978; Cohler, 1982). Results on the respondents were mixed: twelve ranked high on coherence; eight intermediate; and ten low. On reconciliation, twelve ranked high; nine intermediate; and nine low. Coherence and reconciliation were found to be strongly interrelated (.74). The most positive ranking was to be high on both; ten rated high on both.

The themes of coherence and reconciliation were notably not associated with either HIV-serostatus or relationship status. Several HIV-positive men conveyed a strong sense of coherence in their self-appraisals, stating that HIV had provided additional focus and meaning to their lives (Hopcke, 1992).

Both single and coupled men experienced coherence and reconciliation. Whereas single men spoke of the importance of achieving self-sufficiency as a unifying theme in their lives, coupled men described how their relationships provided them with an overaching sense of personal identity. Some men felt that their partnerships provided an antidote to difficulties with self-acceptance (Kertzner, 1999).

Some of the negatives experienced in Kertzner's (1999) sample also had a positive side. When coherence was low, the men felt that life did not turn out as expected or that there were psychological and social dislocations. However, some made sense of this as part of their story of transformation. In terms of reconciliation, many men described false starts or delays in their adult lives such as fledgling heterosexual relationships or the subordination of career development as they explored and consolidated their sexual orientation. The most common regret, voiced by eight men, was a delay in self-acceptance of their gay identity. The study participants articulated different perspectives on delays or missteps in their life histories. The most positive perspective was an appreciation of mistakes as a necessary part of growth, and some did not believe in regrets.

Midlife Lesbian and Gay Persons

The eighty lesbian (thirty-nine) and gay persons (forty-one), all over the age of fifty, from a midwestern metropolitan area studied by Quam and Whitford (1992), reported current health as good or excellent. Most other health data on both midlife and older gay persons focuses on the negative health status of HIV/AIDS (versus the health positives that have been reported in this chapter).

In terms of psychological development, according to Erik Erikson (1980, 1982), adults should resolve three stages: intimacy versus isolation, generativity versus stagnation, and integrity versus despair. These stages present similar challenges for LGBT persons, but they may resolve the issues in different ways than do heterosexual persons.

Generativity is an expected positive development in midlife, although many younger and older adults are also concerned with the welfare of the next generation (Hostetler, 2000). Traditional definitions of generativity include guiding the next generation and making a contribution to future generations (Ryff, 1984; Vaillant, 1993). These tasks are demonstrated in personal commitments to make life better for future generations and can take the form of political and social activism, careers in teaching and social work, activism, mentoring, public health, envrionmentalism and conservation, or volunteering in social or political organizations that assist others (Hostelter, 2000; Isay, 1996). Contributions to future generations of LGBT persons can also be achieved by participating in the struggle for civil rights for these persons (Humphreys & Quam, 1998). Parenthood is also a common generative source for LGBT persons. They may have their own children, live with partners who have children, serve as foster or adoptive parents (Cohler et al., 1998), or they may reach out to assist other children such as nieces, nephews, and godchildren, or children of lesbian and gay friends (Humphreys & Quam, 1998).

Many LGBT persons give back to the community by working as advocates, activists, and volunteers in HIV/AIDS service organizations ("Homosexuals Said to Face," 1994). Some midlife persons were leaders in the creation of services for gay persons with HIV/AIDS (Kimmel & Sang, 1995). Aside from providing services for these persons and caring for them, generativity also includes efforts to curtail the epidemic for the next generation. Lesbians adopted their own mission in breast cancer prevention and concern for the health of the next generation of lesbians (Cohler et al., 1998). Many lesbians also participate in caregiving for gay persons with HIV/AIDS, fundraising for research on HIV/AIDS, and more services those with HIV/AIDS (L. B. Brown et al., 1997).

SUMMARY

One of the major stereotypes of lesbian and gay persons is that they will end up in old age alone, lonely, and depressed. Most of the research refutes this picture, especially for those who are affirmative and reject the heterosexist ideology. Older lesbian and gay persons are as well adjusted as their heterosexual counterparts and younger lesbian and gay persons. Various variables have been looked at as possibly influencing well-adjusted older lesbian and gay persons such as independence, sex-gender role flexibility, and satisfaction with sexual identity. Both mental health and physical health are reported to be good if not better than good. Midlife for many lesbian and gay persons is the best time of life. Except for the HIV/AIDs crisis that is still taking lives, physical health is also reported to be good or better among midlife lesbian and gay persons. The devastation of HIV/AIDS, however, has overshadowed much of the potential positives for those who have lost partners or are coping with their own diagnosis.

Chapter 6

Downturns of Aging

Although there are important differences such as heterosexism, lesbian and gay persons confront many of the same concerns that heterosexual persons confront when they are aging (Adelman, 1990; Kehoe, 1989; J. A. Lee, 1987; Minnigerode & Adelman, 1978; Ehrenberg, 1996). These issues can be categorized as psychological, economics and housing, and health.

PSYCHOLOGICAL ISSUES

Negative Internalizations from Ageism

Ageism is the devaluing of, exclusion of, or discrimination against persons because of age. Older lesbian and gay persons also experience ageism within LGBT communities in which being old is less attractive, less important, less useful, and less worthy of attention and resources (Cahill et al., 2000). In the past, younger persons were introduced by older lesbian and gay persons into safe social circles where they learned about supportive persons and professionals. Beginning in the late 1960s, however, the young began to form their own social, political, and economic organizations especially in large- and mid-sized metropolitan areas as well as in college and university towns (Claes & Moore, 2000). Now, older lesbian and gay persons often feel ignored or dismissed by younger lesbian and gay persons. They are also excluded from community discussions and issues pertinent to them and absent from the mainstream GLBT political agenda (Cahill et al., 2000). What happens psychologically with ageism is an internalization of outside perceptions as one thinks of oneself as being less desirable, capable, important and, being on the way out (B. E. Jones, 2001).

Not all lesbian and gay persons are troubled by ageism. For example, most of the gay persons (ages forty to fifty-five) studied by Kertzner (1999) experienced coming to terms with their sexual identity as more emotionally salient than the incremental process of aging. The experience of aging was far less difficult than establishing a gay identity in their twenties or, for some, their thirties. Most did not report psychological distress associated with getting older.

Distress from Victimization

While most older lesbian and gay persons studied by Grossman et al. (2001) appear to have developed some resilience to the stress related to their sexual identity, they still experience distress. Most striking is the distress from victimization based on sexual identity, with almost two-thirds (63 percent) having experienced verbal abuse, and more than one-quarter (29 percent) reporting threats of physical violence. More than one-quarter (29 percent) also reported being victimized by someone who threatened to disclose their sexual orientation. As indicated by Herek et al. (1999), stigma-based personal attacks on LGB adults are more deleterious to their mental health than other types of attacks.

Loneliness

Loneliness is a major worry for both heterosexual and lesbian and gay persons, particularly as they become among the old-old. Loneliness was experienced by some of the older lesbian and gay participants studied by D'Augelli et al. (2001). More than one-quarter (27 percent) reported lacking companionship, and 13 percent said they felt isolated. Age and loneliness, however, were unrelated. Berger (1996) found that older and younger gay persons did not differ in self-perceived loneliness. Only about one-third of the older gay persons lived alone; two-fifths lived with a lover and the rest with roommates or family members. Many studies have also found that loneliness is no more frequent among older lesbians and gay persons than it is among older heterosexuals (e.g., Berger, 1996; Wahler & Gabbay, 1997).

Neither time spent with other lesbian and gay persons or involvement with lesbian and gay organizations was related to loneliness in the D'Augelli et al. (2001) study. Nor were there significant differences between loneliness and sex-gender or sexual orientations. A significant positive correlation was found between loneliness and household income; the more income, the less loneliness. Also, the more persons in one's support network, the less loneliness. Those living with a partner were less lonely. Those who experienced more victimization experienced more loneliness.

Many of the older lesbian and gay persons studied by Grossman et al. (2001) endorsed the view that individuals are responsible for their loneliness. Slightly more than half (52 percent) of the respondents agreed or strongly agreed that loneliness is a persons' own fault. Feeling responsible was not related to sexual orientation, living with a partner or living alone, household income, number of people in one's support network, time spent with other lesbian or gay persons, or involvement in lesbian or gay organizations.

Despair

Integrity versus despair is the major challenge that Erikson (1980) proposed for those at older ages. Integrity means accepting who one is and what one's life has been. Some of the older gay persons studied by Kertzner (1999) were unable to accept their lives and appeared to be experiencing despair. For those who experience despair, a common form is a sense that much of their life has been wasted because of their discomfort with their sexual orientation. This may be magnified by severed relationships because parents, siblings, children, marital partners, and friends did not accept them (Humphreys & Quam, 1998).

For several older gay persons studied by Kertzner (1999), becoming middle-aged adults exacerbated feelings of missed opportunities to raise children, pursue career aspirations that were deferred earlier in life, or experience success in long-term relationships. An additional three men felt stuck in their current midlife situation. They cited poor prospects of earning more money, difficulty forming intimate relationships, and increasing concerns about their desirability to younger partners. They experienced a need to catch up with peers whom they judged as enjoying more successful and full lives. These men reported lengthy periods of depression or alcohol use in their young adulthood, which they felt played a part in lagging behind peers in life fulfillment.

Some of the men had a sense of never recovering from earlier errors and described a pervasive sense of regret about not seizing opportunities to advance careers or pursue relationships in young adulthood, making impulsive decisions that they believed had long-lasting detrimental effects on their adult lives, or not coming out sooner to parents. In middle age, they perceived less opportunity to overcome previous failures and described greater worry that negative life experiences such as romantic or sexual rejection would happen again (Kertzner, 1999).

Suicidal Ideation

The older lesbian and gay persons studied by D'Augelli et al. (2001) had not often considered suicide. Overall, 10 percent said they considered suicide sometimes or often; 13 percent reported a suicide attempt, generally between the ages of twenty-two and fifty-nine. About a quarter of attempts (27 percent) were made before participants were twenty-one years old, 69 percent between the ages of twenty-two and fifty-nine, and 4 percent at or after age sixty. Lower lifetime suicidal ideation was predicted by less negative feelings about one's sexual orientation, less loneliness, and a higher percent of persons who knew one's orientation. More suicidal thinking was attributed to conflicts about sexual orientation. Gay men reported more suicidal thoughts related to sexual orientation than did lesbians. Those who experienced suicidal thoughts also reported being lonelier and having less control over their loneliness. They were lower in self-esteem. They abused alcohol and drugs more. They were less physically healthy and had worse cognitive functioning. Parents had more often thought about suicide over their lifetimes than nonparents. More parents (19 percent) reported suicide attempts than nonparents (11 percent). Those who reported a mental disability had more than twice as many past suicide attempts (26 percent) as those who did not report a mental disability.

LOSS AND BEREAVEMENT

Loss is an integral part of the aging process, be it physical or psychological. The loss of a long-time partner can be especially difficult for older lesbian and gay persons. Others may not know of the severity of the loss if a relationship was never defined as a partnership. The partner may feel it necessary to hide the grieving process from others so as to hide the relationship. It may also mean the loss of material possessions or financial supports that were previously considered joint ownership (Fullmer, 1995; Fullmer et al., 1999; Shenk, 1998). Community programs serving HIV/AIDS patients might be possible avenues for offering sensitive, supportive grief counseling (Claes & Moore, 2000).

ECONOMICS AND HOUSING ISSUES

Economics

Older LGBT persons are more likely to live alone and lack family support networks. They may experience poverty or economic insecurity at higher rates than heterosexual counterparts (Cahill et al., 2000). Although this is changing in a few states and cities, the lack of marriage rights and spousal benefits for most couples can create serious financial hardships, especially if one's partner dies. The surviving partner may be forced out of the home shared with a partner (Claes & Moore, 2000).

Several federal programs and laws do not apply to same sex-gender couples as they do to married heterosexual couples. For example, Social Security pays survivor benefits to widows and widowers, but not to the surviving same sex-gender life partner of someone who dies. Married heterosexual partners are eligible for Social Security spousal benefits, which can allow them to attain half their partner's Social Security benefit if it is larger than their own benefit. Unmarried same sex-gender partners in life-long relationships are not eligible for these benefits. Medicare regulations protect the assets and homes of heterosexual married partners when the other partner enters a nursing home or long-term care facility. No such protections are offered to same sex-gender partners. Tax laws and other regulations of 401(k)s and pensions also discriminate against same sex-gender partners (Cahill et al., 2000).

If legal marriage becomes more prevalent for lesbian and gay persons, the situation discussed here will change because they will have the same rights as heterosexual couples. This includes:

Tax Benefits

- Filing joint income tax returns with the IRS and state taxing authorities
- Creating a "family partnership" under federal tax laws, which allows you to divide business income among family members

Estate Planning Benefits

- Inheriting a share of your spouse's estate
- Receiving an exemption from both estate taxes and gift taxes for all property you give or leave to your spouse
- Creating life estate trusts that are restricted to married couples, including Qualified Terminal Interest Property (QTIP) Trusts, Qualified Domestic (QDOT) Trusts, and marital deduction trusts
- Obtaining priority if a conservator needs to be appointed for your spouse—that is, someone to make financial and/or medical decisions on your spouse's behalf

Government Benefits

- Receiving Social Security, Medicare, and disability benefits for spouses
- Receiving veterans' and military benefits for spouses, such as those for education, medical care, or special loans
- Receiving public assistance benefits

Employment Benefits

- Obtaining insurance benefits through a spouse's employer
- Taking family leave to care for your spouse during an illness
- Receiving wages, workers' compensation, and retirement plan benefits for a deceased spouse
- Taking bereavement leave if your spouse or one of your spouse's close relatives dies

Medical Benefits

- Visiting your spouse in a hospital intensive care unit or during restricted visiting hours in other parts of a medical facility

- Making medical decisions for your spouse if he or she becomes incapacitated and unable to express wishes for treatment

Death Benefits

- Consenting to after-death examinations and procedures
- Making burial or other final arrangements

Family Benefits

- Filing for stepparent or joint adoption
- Applying for joint foster care rights
- Receiving equitable division of property if you divorce
- Receiving spousal or child support, child custody, and visitation if you divorce

Housing Benefits

- Living in neighborhoods zoned for "families only"
- Automatically renewing leases signed by your spouse

Consumer Benefits

- Receiving family rates for health, homeowners', auto, and other types of insurance
- Receiving tuition discounts and permission to use school facilities
- Other consumer discounts and incentives offered only to married couples or families

Other Legal Benefits and Protections

- Suing a third person for wrongful death of your spouse and loss of consortium (loss of intimacy)
- Suing a third person for offenses that interfere with the success of your marriage, such as alienation of affection and criminal conversation (these laws are available in only a few states)
- Claiming the marital communications privilege, which means a court can't force you to disclose the contents of confidential communications between you and your spouse during your marriage

- Receiving crime victims' recovery benefits if your spouse is the victim of a crime
- Obtaining domestic violence protection orders
- Obtaining immigration and residency benefits for noncitizen spouse
- Visiting rights in jails and other places where visitors are restricted to immediate family (Nolo, 2004)

Housing

The main reason for LGBT affordable communities is so this population: can live among others similar to themselves and receive services from an understanding agency; can live without fear of harassment or neglect because of their sexual identities; and can have a comfortable place to grow old. Many of these persons want to remain in their own communities with friends and loved ones (Human Rights, 2000).

At the federal level, Housing and Urban Development (HUD) rules do not deny housing to nonheterosexual persons but this inclusion is not based on law and may not be followed according to the preferences of particular administration. Nothing protects transgender persons as they are never protected by these rules; only one state offers housing or public accommodation protection for transgender persons (Van de Meide, 2000). Specific housing needs and availability are discussed in Chapter 8.

HEALTH CARE SYSTEM

Although health is good for many midlife and older LGB persons, they fear illness and the insensitivity of health care providers. Many LGBT persons have limited access to health care and often experience discrimination and bias. Many LGBT persons are uninsured, underinsured, unaware of, or geographically too far from an LGBT-friendly source of care (Mail, 2002). Limited access to needed services was a substantial problem for midlife lesbians (Bradford & Ryan, 1991). Limited financial resources affect both essential and preventive health care. A little more than a quarter of these women had no health insurance. On the other hand, if the health problems were serious, such as thyroid problems or high blood pressure, they were generally receiving care.

While urban areas have seen improved access to specialized care for LGBT persons, rural areas with low numbers of LGBT consumers are still unlikely to provide knowledgeable, compassionate care (Meyer, 2001). Butler and Hope (1999) reported that twelve of the twenty-four midlife lesbians they interviewed who lived in Maine had disclosed their sexual identity to their health providers. Eight reported discrimination as lesbians in accessing health care and eight as women. Six had no health insurance. Poverty and lack of health insurance were the primary obstacles to receiving good health care. Poverty faced by nearly a third of the lesbians resulted from limited economic opportunities in rural areas, age and gender discrimination in employment, and strict eligibility requirements for disability benefits. Distance from health care providers was another obstacle.

The Gay and Lesbian Medical Association and the Center for LGBT Health at Columbia University have identified a number of major structural concerns related to GLBT health overall, including: lack of a coordinated public health infrastructure to support and direct funded initiatives on GLBT health; institutional barriers to quality health services, such as denial of benefits to same sex-gender partners or children by insurers and employers; and barriers to communication between health care providers and LGBT consumers. Same sex-gender partners have no say in the disposition of an incapacitated partner in most cities unless advanced directives such as health care proxies and powers of attorney have been completed (Karp, 2000). Emergency rooms and inpatient units also restrict or deny access to partners and nonbiological parents (Dean et al., 2000).

Aside from the systemic issues, many medical practitioners either openly or secretly hold negative attitudes regarding LGBT persons. Although there have been changes in the past twenty years, studies continue to show that health care providers are still reluctant to treat lesbian and gay persons and even worse, are hostile and demeaning toward them (Stevens, 1994). Heterosexist practices may be conveyed through nonverbal communication such as avoiding eye contact, maintaining distance, or refraining from touching a patient who is lesbian or gay. The message is imparted that the provider is uncomfortable with or disapproving of these persons. "We don't treat your kind here" may not be said, but nevertheless communicated (Claes & Moore, 2000). Most members (88 percent) of the Gay and Lesbian Medical Association had heard colleagues disparage lesbian and gay patients, 67 percent knew of associates who denied care, and more than half (52 percent) observed colleagues reducing care or denying care to patients because of sexual orientation (Schatz & O'Hanlan, 1994). As late as 1991, one in seven family practice and internal medicine residents still considered homosexuality a mental disorder (Hayward & Weissfeld, 1993; Harrison, 1996).

Many lesbian and gay persons reported insensitive physicians who were not knowledgeable about LGBT health risks and needs and did not disclose pertinent information about treatments or prevention (Schatz & O'Hanlan, 1994; Trippet & Bain, 1992). Many of these consumers do not disclose their sexual orientation to health care providers because they do not feel comfortable doing so, or they fear receiving substandard care (Cochran & Mays, 1988; White & Dull, 1997). Many Web resources for health knowledge and affirmative health practitioners are available. One of the most extensive resources is the Gay and Lesbian Medical Association Web site (http://www.gima.org/).

Older lesbian and gay persons may avoid seeking medical care because of a fear that their sexual identity will be discovered by doctors, home attendants, social workers, hospital staff, or visiting nurses. They may feel that revealing a lesbian or gay identity is not important if it means receiving biased or inferior services (Altman, 1999). As noted earlier, these persons grew up when acknowledgment of their sexual identity to a family physician or psychiatrist could result in diagnosis of mental illness, and possibly institutionalization. This age cohort was forced to create a hidden life and many have continued to live this way (Fassinger, 1991). Anecdotal reports indicate other forms of discrimination against older lesbian and gay persons such as forced separation of long-term partners in nursing homes, prejudicial comments made by staff or other residents of retirement communities, and failure of community or senior centers to provide information or support on gay or lesbian specific issues (Gewirtzman & Kaelber, 2000).

Partners are often not officially recognized in the medical system although they may have lived together in a stable relationship for many years. Where life partners are not explicitly designated as the person in charge or where such declarations are ignored, they can be excluded from all aspects of the decision-making process regarding treatment of a partner. If opposed to the relationship, blood relatives may step in and control treatment options, visitations, finances, transfer to other institutions, and discharge planning. Hospitals, nursing homes, inpatient hospice programs, retirement homes, assisted living facilities, and adult day care programs may directly or indirectly seek to create barriers between life partners. Staff often discourage or obstruct outward signs of affection such as hugging or holding of hands through comments, indirect communications, or stated "policies" (Claes & Moore, 2000).

Transgender persons are at an even greater risk for poor quality care. Doctors often refuse to treat them, use inappropriate pronouns, or fail to provide necessary care (Lombardi, 2001). Because they may be insensitive to the difference between sex-gender identity and sexual orientation they might assume that transgender persons have the same health care needs as LGB patients (Garbo, 2000). There may also be lack of sensitivity to the differences in identities experienced, and physical form which creates different needs and strategies. Attention is not directed to the actual experiences of transgender persons (Lombardi, 2001). This lack of sensitivity can adversely influence whether these persons will access and stay in treatment (JSI Research and Training Institute, 2000). The American Public Health Association's 1999 resolution stated the need for health care providers and to provide transgender persons with culturally relevant and sensitive treatment and resources (APHA policy statement, 2000). An increasing number of books and articles exist on transgender persons which specify their needs (Lombardi, 2001).

Alzheimer's disease and related dementia has profound effects on the lives of family, friends, and the community (Alzheimer's Association, 1995). In addition to providing interventions for patients, social services agencies can be of help to the caregivers. The New York City chapter of the Alzheimer's Association, in conjunction with SAGE, recently established a support group for LGBT caregivers of others with dementia (J. A. Levine & Altman, 2002). W. R. Moore (2002) described the development of a telephone support group for older lesbian and gay persons caring for life partners with Alzheimer's disease or other severe disorders in a rural, eleven-county area of western North Carolina. Two proven human service delivery models—support groups and telephone conferencing—were combined. The group met for six sessions and dealt with a number of themes including legal and financial issues, anticipatory grief, and the struggle with closure. A postgroup questionnaire showed that the sense of isolation was reduced for group members, their social support system increased, and their determination to continue in the caregiver role and to keep the life partner in the home as long as possible was affirmed.

SUMMARY

Lesbian and gay persons confront the same downturns in older age as heterosexual persons. The main difference is the heterosexism that they face in social and medical services. Internalized ageism affects all older persons, but lesbian and gay persons may be able to cope with it better since they have been coping with heterosexism since coming out. Some lesbian and gay persons experience other downturns including victimization because of sexual orientation, loneliness, despair, and suicidal thinking. The loss of a long-term partner is especially difficult. Because most lesbian and gay persons do not get the benefits that heterosexual persons get from legal marriage, social security, tax laws, and so on, they may have more economic hardships when older. They may also lose their residence when a partner dies if protections are not in place. It is usual to encounter heterosexism from medical staffs when lesbian and gay persons need services in the health or social services systems. This situation is even more difficult for transgender persons.

PART IV:
PRACTICE WITH MIDLIFE AND OLDER LGBT PERSONS

Chapter 7

Changes in Diagnostics, Treatments, and Human Services

"Homosexuality" was viewed as a sin during much of the nineteenth century (Gonsiorek, 1982a). Later it was medicalized (Bérubé, 1990; Rosenberg & Golden, 1992), and by the early part of the twentieth century it was viewed as a mental illness (Morin, 1977). Mainstream psychological practice, based on psychoanalytic theories, equated "homosexuality" with pathology (Lewes, 1988). Although Freud (1949) did not think "homosexual" persons were pathologically impaired, his view was not accepted by many of his earlier and later followers. Instead, they viewed "homosexuality" as a serious deviation that negatively affects one's total social functioning (Bayer, 1987). These negative views and attitudes, however, were not based on dispassionate scientific research, none of which then existed (Herek, 1991). Only in the late 1940s and early 1950s did empirically based research begin to emerge on "homosexuality," and to strongly challenge the view that it was a mental illness. In the 1960s, a special committee of the British legislature concluded that "homosexual" persons were well adjusted and recommended the repeal of British laws that prohibited same sex-gender sexual behavior between consenting adults (Wolfenden, 1963).

The most sensational research results in the United States came from a pioneering study on gay persons reported in 1957. When she was a young psychologist at the University of California at Los Angeles, the National Institute of Mental Health awarded Evelyn Hooker a grant for a longitudinal study. The purpose was to compare the personality structure and adjustment of thirty heterosexual men and thirty gay men. All the respondents were matched for age, intelligence, and educational level. No one was in therapy. The gay respondents came from community organizations instead of being patients in psychoanalysis or prisoners as in earlier studies. Hooker used the standard battery of tools available to American psychologists in the 1950s to assess personality and adjustment. This included projective techniques (Rorschach Ink Blot Test, Thematic Apperception Test, and Make-a-Picture-Story Test), attitude scales, and intensive life history interviews (Bullough, 1994b). At the time it was unthinkable that a "homosexual" could be psychologically healthy, but Hooker (1957) concluded from the results of the research that same sex-gender sexual orientation was not inherently pathological. The clinicians, unaware of any respondent's sexual orientation, could not identify which profiles were those of the gay respondents and which were those of the heterosexual respondents. Using a five-point scale, they classified two-thirds of each group as in the three highest categories of adjustment (average or better). Most of the gay men were happy and productive and some of them were functioning at superior levels.

Hooker's work was followed by more than 100 additional empirical studies focused on the mental health of both lesbian and gay persons (e.g., Adelman, 1977; Freedman, 1971; N. L. Thompson, McCandless, & Strickland, 1971). Almost every study confirmed Hooker's basic finding that few significant differences existed between lesbian and gay samples and samples of heterosexual women and men in mental health. Enough studies were done with acceptable designs and samples to show a clear and consistent pattern: "homosexuality" in and of itself is unrelated to maladjustment or psychopathology (Gonsiorek, 1982b). Bisexual persons were also found to not be pathological or psychologically maladjusted (e.g., Masters & Johnson, 1979; Nurius, 1983; Zinik, 1985). Research has also demonstrated that the behavior and identity of transgender persons do not impair their lives (Lombardi, 1999).

BATTLES AND VICTORIES

Lesbian and Gay Persons

These studies showing that "homosexuality" was not a mental illness did not quickly change the classification of "homosexuality" as a mental illness in the American Psychiatric Association's *Diagnostic and Statistical Manual of Mental Disorders*. It took two decades of struggle and three years of intense challenge by activists in the Gay Liberation Movement and allies in the American Psychiatric Association (APA) to get this classification eliminated (e.g., Barr & Catts, 1974; Green, 1972; Marmor, 1972). On December 15, 1973, the APA board of trustees unanimously voted to remove "homosexuality" from its official list of psychiatric disorders (e.g., Adam, 1987). Hence, the diagnostic category of "homosexuality" was not present in the 1980 edition of APA's *Diagnostic and Statistical Manual of Mental Disorders,* Third Edition (DSM-III). Yet a new diagnostic category appeared—"sexual orientation disturbance" (later called "ego-dystonic homosexuality"). This category was supposedly applicable to persons who felt upset with having a same-sex sexual orientation and wanted to change it. Lesbian and gay psychiatrists, psychologists, and social workers pressured the APA to remove this category, and in the revised third edition (DSM-III-R) in 1987, it was absent (Morin & Rothblum, 1991; T. S. Stein, 1993).

Transgender Persons

Transgender persons are still fighting the DSM battles that lesbian and gay persons fought in the 1970s (Gagné et al., 1997). Although there was no mention of transgender or transsexual in the 1994 DSM-IV, the diagnostic category gender identity disorder (GID) was and is still present (Denny, 1999). This category applies to a person who experiences "cross-sex identification, feelings of discomfort and inappropriateness in one's assigned [sex-] gender role, the absence of a physical intersex condition, and impairment in social, occupational, or other arenas of living" (Anderson, 1998, p. 222).

The problem with the GID label is society's refusal to accept a nondualistic view of sex-gender roles. The problem is not the persons who cannot or refuse to fit into dualistic sex-gender roles (Anderson, 1998). Cross-dressing (by heterosexual or bisexual males) is also still categorized as "transvestic fetishism" although a growing body of evidence shows that cross-dressing is not a mental disorder (Cole et al., 2000; Denny, 1997, 1999). Transgender activists want to reduce the domination of mental health professionals over the lives of transgender persons (International Conference on Transgender Law, 1994). They also want both GID and transvestic fetishism removed from the DSM (Cole et al., 2000).

Transgender persons also want the standards for sexual reassignment surgery (SRS) modified. Harry Benjamin and his associates provided groundbreaking arguments for sex-gender reassignment for persons in a 1966 publication, *The Transsexual Phenomenon* (Denny, 2002). However, the updated 1998 Standards of Care by the Harry Benjamin International Gender Dysphoria Association narrowed the definition of "transsexualism" and thereby restricted those who could qualify for SRS. The Benjamin model also acknowledged only two sex-genders, leaving out anyone who wants to live outside this binary construction (S. B. Levine et al., 1998).

Persons who felt that their sex-gender identity did not match their biological sex began to disclose to each other at the 1985 International Foundation for Gender Education forum in Boston. They also revealed that they did not conform to the Benjamin criteria for transsexuals or transvestites. These meetings and disclosures led to the development of an alternative model in the 1990s, the transgender model (Cole et al., 2000). This is now the accepted model in the transgender community, It encourages acceptance of an infinite number of sex-gender identities and ways of life. Revisions are underway in the Benjamin criteria that reflect this view (Denny, 1999).

Intersex Persons

An intersex person is born with both male and female physical characteristics. There are a variety of intersex conditions. Some intersex persons can match their physical situation with the life they lead while others experience considerable difficulty doing this (M. Diamond, 2002). The genitals of many intersex persons were altered at birth to fit either a male or female sex-gender identity, but this alteration may not fit with one's inner feelings later (Israel & Tarver, 1997). In the 1990s, intersex persons began to oppose the medical regulation of and mutilation of their bodies. There is no essential reason for surgical alteration in infancy as ambiguous genitals are neither painful nor harmful to health. The surgeries are destructive and often debilitating to the patients and serve only a cosmetic purpose (Chase, 2002).

A peer-support network of intersex persons grew into the Intersex Society of North America (ISNA) (http://www.isna.org). This organization was formed in response to individual cases of trauma

caused by surgeries. The goals are to reform the treatment of intersex persons, to limit the practice of surgical interventions to those
that are medically necessary, and to limit surgeries performed on
children purely for the sake of aesthetics (Lombardi, 2001). It is
best for the child to have the say, after puberty, in how he or she is allowed to live (M. Diamond & Sigmundson, 1997).

OPPRESSIVE TREATMENTS
OF LESBIAN AND GAY PERSONS

Another issue for lesbian and gay persons was the prescribed
treatments to cure them from their "homosexuality." Often, punitive
and coercive treatments were applied in asylums after commitment
by families or the criminal justice system. Treatments included in-
duced seizures, nausea-inducing drugs, electric shock, aversion
therapy, "covert sensitization," masturbation while viewing pictures
of a nude woman, lobotomy, castration, hysterectomies, implanta-
tion of "normal" testes, untested drugs, and supplementation of various hormones. Although psychotherapy was more humane, the
goal was the same—to cure the "homosexual" patient of the disease
of "homosexuality" (D'Emilio, 1983; Haldeman, 1994; Silverstein,
1991, 1996). The most common psychotherapy approaches were
psychoanalysis and behavior modification, but they did not result in
any "cures" (e.g., Curran & Parr, 1957; Freund, 1977; Halderman,
1994: Mayerson & Lief, 1965; Mintz, 1996).

No treatment can change persons who have exclusive attractions
to others of the same sex-gender (Green, 2003; Isay, 1990). Even
when persons claim to be cured from "homosexuality," they only
control their sexual behavior. Sexual attractions to others of the
same sex-gender are still present (Conrad & Wincze, 1976; Rangaswami, 1982). Even for those who report happy marriages, same
sex-gender fantasies persist (Birk, 1980). Eventually, adverse pub-
licity about the treatments to change sexual orientation and the research showing that same sex-gender sexual orientation is not
pathological led to the reduction of these attempts to change a person's sexual orientation (Dynes & S. Donaldson, 1992).

THE NEW AFFIRMATIVE PRACTICE

Professional organizations representing human services practitioners no longer endorse the oppressive treatments just reviewed. After "homosexuality" was removed as a diagnostic category from the American Psychiatric Association's *Diagnostic and Statistical Manual of Mental Disorders* in 1973, one by one, these organizations passed resolutions declaring that "homosexuality" was no longer to be labeled a mental illness. They also directed their members to deliver unbiased services to LGBT persons and to advocate to end discrimination directed at them. Beginning in the early 1970s, lesbian and gay counseling centers opened in major urban cities such as New York and Seattle and provided "gay affirmative" services. The affirmative approach to practice is not a technique but a frame of reference (Malyon, 1981-1982). It is a moral practice (Hartman & Laird, 1998) that encourages lesbian and gay persons to accept and value their sexual identities and sexual attractions. An affirmative focus has also developed for bisexual persons (e.g., Matteson, 1996a; Nichols, 1988) and for transgender persons (e.g., Emerson & Rosenfeld, 1996; C. Rosenfeld & Emerson, 1998).

HUMAN SERVICES TODAY

LGB persons show no greater "maladjustment" than heterosexual persons and they show social, psychological, and political resiliency while living in oppressive societies (Appleby & Anastas, 1998). Yet they seek services in every helping field (L. S. Brown, 1996). Both lesbian and gay persons who use "therapy" do so more often and are in "therapy" for longer periods of time compared to heterosexual persons (Liddle, 1997). In a national sample of 1,633 lesbians surveyed by Sorensen and Roberts (1997), about half (50 percent) had seen a "therapist" more than twice. Compared to 29 percent of heterosexual women, more than two-thirds (78 percent) of lesbians saw a mental health professional in samples studied by Morgan (1992). In another survey by Bernhard and Applegate (1999), lesbians were significantly more likely (86 percent) to report seeing a practitioner at some time than were heterosexual women (54 percent). Little data exist about utilization of therapy specifically by older lesbian and gay persons. Bradford and Ryan (1987) found that the oldest age group in their sample of lesbians (fifty-five years and above) saw practitioners less frequently than did women ages twenty-five to fifty-four, but slightly more frequently than women ages seventeen to twenty-four.

Fortunately for lesbian and gay clients, services have greatly improved over recent years (Liddle, 1999). Most lesbian and gay clients (86 percent) studied by M.A. Jones and Gabriel (1999) reported that "therapy" had a positive effect on their lives; 50 percent felt "very positive" about "therapy"; and 33 percent felt that "therapy" had "saved their lives." Respondents indicated in ratings on a ten-point scale that they felt liked by the practitioner (7.8), felt respected by the practitioner (7.8), felt understood by the practitioner (7.2), and felt accepted by the practitioner (7.9).

ONGOING HETEROSEXIST ATTITUDES IN PRACTICE

Some practitioners still think of LGB clients as abnormal, believe they can change their sexual orientation, lack knowledge about their concerns, and lack understanding of the negative effects of heterosexist oppression on every aspect of the practice process (Berkman & Zinberg, 1997; E. Cramer, 1997; Garnets, Hancock, Cochran, Goodchilds, & Peplau, 1991; McHenry & Johnson, 1993). Heterosexist attitudes displayed in practice can range from overt to liberal and all are hurtful and unacceptable (Riddle, 1996).

The most extreme level of heterosexist attitudes is called *repulsion*. Here, practitioners view same sex-gender sexual orientation as a crime against nature, and LGB persons as sick, sinful, and immoral (Riddle, 1996). These practitioners feel superior and are judgmental, condescending, and disrespectful to LGB persons generally and as clients (S.M. Donaldson, 1998). They mainly want to change their sexual orientations.

Several other levels of heterosexist attitudes, identified by Riddle (1996), include:

- *Pity:* Practitioners view heterosexuality as preferable to any other sexual orientation. Persons who cannot change their lesbian, gay, or bisexual sexual orientation or seem born that way should be pitied.

- *Tolerance:* Practitioners tolerate same sex-gender or bisexual sexual orientations as just a phase of adolescent development that eventually will be outgrown. These practitioners treat those who do not outgrow this "phase" or are "immature" in their development with the protectiveness and indulgence one might apply to a young child.
- *Acceptance:* Practitioners say they accept LGB persons. Thinking that they have to accept them, however, implies that these clients have a "problem."
- *Liberal:* Practitioners are friendly with LGB persons but have not thought beyond this to how they are still biased. They display heterosexist bias, for example, when they take for granted the privilege associated with heterosexual status. In addition, while they disapprove of overt bias and prejudice they feel uncomfortable with overt displays of affection between same sex-gender persons or with the ambiguity of transgender or bisexual identifications.

All these practices are harmful to LGB clients. Unless practitioners can abandon prior assumptions and myths about LGB persons (Laird, 1995, 1996) and comply with standards of ethical practice with these clients, they should never provide any kind of services for them. Training sessions on heterosexism and bias toward LGB persons might change attitudes if biased practitioners are willing and ready to change (e.g., DiAngelo, 1997; Sears and Williams, 1997).

Institutional denial of the specific needs of LGBT clients also occurs. Many administrators of social services agencies seem to not realize that LGBT persons have specific needs, and they see no point in developing affirmative programs specifically for LGBT clients. They may argue, for example, that these clients can explore relationship and family issues in any of the agency's dating, relationship, or family groups, although these groups are focused on heterosexual and nontransgender persons (Ball, 1994; Hancock, 1995).

Most LGB clients are well aware of institutional denial of their needs and the negative attitudes held by mental health and health professionals, as well as those of the general public (Rothblum, 1994). They have assessed their environments all their lives for signs of prejudice, rejection, hatred, or violence. They note cues via voice or mannerism, awkwardness, defensiveness, hesitancy, hostility, distance, disapproval, contempt, or outright rejection (L. S. Brown, 1989; Fassinger, 1991; M. Pope, 1997). When they perceive that practitioners hold negative views, they can experience greater psychological distress following social services than they experienced before services began (Fassinger, 1991). The openness and trust LGBT clients have for their practitioners will diminish, a situation that is difficult to later correct (Messing, Schoenberg, & Stephens, 1983-1984; M. Pope, 1997). Some clients prematurely terminate because they think that the practitioner will terminate services with them (Alexander, 1998). Others terminate after one session because of unhelpful behaviors by the practitioner (Liddle, 1996).

Unfortunately, practitioners across all disciplines in human services receive little or no education about issues pertinent to LGBT populations (Buhrke & Douce, 1991; Mackelprang, Ray, & Hernandez- Peck, 1996), much less assistance in changing preconceived notions. This is still the case even though codes of ethics of human services professions now endorse training and other requirements regarding LGBT persons.

REQUIREMENTS OF PRACTITIONERS AND SOCIAL SERVICES AGENCIES

If practitioners in human services agencies adhere to a professional code of ethics, they must be affirmative, not oppressive, with LGBT clients. They must serve all clients equitably. As human services organizations provide most of the counseling, case management, and other services for these persons, it is crucial that these organizations insist upon nonjudgmental, affirmative attitudes by their staffs. Practitioners are called upon not only to proclaim accurate views of the mental health of LGBT persons but also to provide compassionate and affirmative services to these persons (Downey & Friedman, 1996; A. S. Hall & Fradkin, 1992). They must continually examine how biases, beliefs, preferences, and convictions shape their attitudes and harm others (Hartman & Laird, 1998). They must take responsibility for attaining both emotional and intellectual competency in their work and interactions with LGBT clients. Ethical dilemmas result if either type of competency is deficient or missing (L. S. Brown, 1996).

Affirmative Emotions and Intellect

Emotional competency involves awareness of personal attitudes and feelings about LGBT persons and willingness to assess emotional readiness to do practice with them. One also has to commit to changing one's biases and prejudices to better offer compassionate and effective services (L. S. Brown, 1996). Self-examination operates on various levels (Markowitz, 1991): What messages do I communicate to LGBT clients about their worth and value? (L. S. Brown, 1995). What assumptions do I make about a client's sexual orientation? Why do I make these assumptions? (Eldridge, 1987). If one is heterosexual, imagine that one's partner is of the same sex-gender. What feelings does this arouse? Fear? Shame? (Hartman & Laird, 1998). At another level, A. S. Hall and Fradkin (1992) posed these questions: "Would I feel very comfortable if a son of mine were gay? Would I feel very comfortable participating in a gay rights march? Will I confront heterosexist jokes when I hear them?" (p. 364).

Perhaps more disturbing to most heterosexual practitioners is this level of question, posed by A. S. Hall and Fradkin (1992): "Am I as comfortable with my ["homosexual"] feelings as my heterosexual feelings?" (p. 364). As discussed in Chapter 1, Kinsey and colleagues confirmed that persons are rarely exclusively heterosexual. Moreover, many persons go through a transient period after puberty when they engage in same sex-gender sexual behavior (Kinsey et al., 1948). In their studies on sexuality, Masters and Johnson (1979) found that same sex-gender erotic imagery was one of the most frequent fantasies reported by the heterosexual group.

A. S. Hall and Fradkin (1992) posed another question: "What homoerotic fantasies, feelings, or behaviors have I had or do I have, and can I appreciate and enjoy these parts of me?" (p. 364). Heterosexual practitioners may not participate in same sex-gender sexual behaviors or fantasize about them, but they may still fear that they are not exclusively heterosexually oriented. It is essential for all practitioners to feel comfortable with their own sexuality and sexual orientation (Cabaj, 1988; Fassinger, 1991).

Emotional competence also involves understanding the affirmative stance on practice and integrating it into one's attitudes and behaviors. The affirmative stance, identified by Riddle (1996), includes three levels:

1. *Support:* Practitioners work to safeguard the rights of LGBT persons because they are aware of the heterosexist climate and the irrational unfairness of it. They support LGBT persons in their efforts to live fuller lives and to experience pride in themselves.
2. *Admiration:* Practitioners admire the courage and strength it takes in society to declare oneself lesbian, gay, bisexual, or transgender.
3. *Appreciation:* Practitioners value the diversity of all persons and see LGBT persons as a valid part of that diversity.

Intellectual competency includes obtaining accurate and scientifically sound information and professional training regarding LGBT persons (L. S. Brown, 1996). Practitioner knowledge of issues specific to lesbian and gay persons is associated with the satisfaction of these clients (Liddle, 1996). Practitioners must become aware of the gaps in their knowledge and seek further training, supervision, and consultation (L. S. Brown, 1996). Aside from knowledge about LGBT persons from literature, practitioners need to let clients tell their story. Literature can help guide questions and exploration of a client's story, but it will not provide information about the unique experiences and meanings of a client's life (Hartman & Laird, 1998). Practitioners must also actively obtain information on suitable and unsuitable practices with LGBT clients (Garnets et al., 1991).

AFFIRMATIVE ENVIRONMENT, LANGUAGE, AND QUESTIONS

From the first moment lesbian and gay clients enter a human services office they evaluate their surroundings for comfort and security (Chernin & Johnson, 2003). It is difficult for LGBT clients to ask for help if the environment is not affirmative (Appleby & Anastas, 1998). Social services agencies should, therefore, provide positive, affirmative environments that communicate a supportive and appreciative atmosphere so clients will feel that they can discuss feelings, experiences, and ideas in a free and open manner (Radkowsky & Siegel, 1997). Affirmative environments include positive written acknowledgment of LGBT persons such as client information forms that offer categories other than single, married, and divorced; the mention of sexual orientation and transgender in statements about working with diverse groups; visible resources such as a pamphlet that addresses concerns of these persons; a logo to indicate that the agency welcomes LGBT clients and that LGBT persons work in the agency (Gruskin, 1999); posters placed on the walls from local or national LGBT organizations; affirmative books, articles, periodicals, and other items focused on LGBT persons displayed on shelves and tables (Barrett, 1998; Croteau and Theil, 1994); affirmative symbols on clothing such as pins or other jewelry (Gruskin, 1999); and staff who know about community resources (Eldridge & Barnett, 1991).

It is important also to make sure that these particular biases are not present: (1) omission bias or ignoring the possibility of a respondent being lesbian or gay; (2) connotation bias, when words with negative connotations are associated with references to minority groups, such as gay and psychopathology or child molester; and (3) contingency bias, when scales used for diagnosing mental illness are placed by scales which are intended to measure characteristics of lesbian and gay persons or refer to lesbian and gay persons amid diagnoses of paranoia, depression, and other forms of mental illness (Chernin & Johnson, 2003).

Respectful, inclusive, and neutral language should be used (Croteau & Morgan, 1989; Croteau & von Destinon, 1994), such as sexual activity versus sexual intercourse; relationship status versus marital status; partner versus spouse; and couples practice versus marital practice (Bernstein, 1992). Instead of asking about marital status on client forms, clients can be asked who is most important to them or who is in their family. This allows clients to complete the forms in the way they choose (Deevey, 1990; Gruskin, 1999; M. Kelly, 1998).

Lesbian and gay clients should also be allowed to state what they call themselves as individuals and as couples. Labels should not be assumed by practitioners. For example, the term *homosexual* is not neutral. It should never be used as it is usually viewed as negative and is too clinical and distancing. Gay persons generally prefer the term gay; for lesbians acceptable terms are less clear-cut. Most of them find lesbian acceptable but some object to this term and prefer to be called gay while others want to avoid that term (Faria, 1997). Couples mostly use the term lover or partner, but husband, wife, roommate, friend, or girlfriend or boyfriend may also be used. Also, a broader definition of family should be incorporated which includes family of origin, children, a partner who may or may not live with the client, and ex-lovers (Ainslie & Feltey, 1991; Hooyman & Lustbader, 1986; Kimmel, 1992).

Similarly, neutral terms should be used in questions as well as use open-ended questions: Who is essential to you? What can you tell me about your relationships? What can you tell me about the persons who are significant in your life? Who are the significant children in your life? (Claes & Moore, 2000; McAllan & Ditillo, 1994). Who would you like to include in discussions about your treatment or your appointments? (Claes & Moore, 2000; Gruskin, 1999; McAllan & Ditillo, 1994.) It is important not to ask questions that assume a client's heterosexuality, now or at any time in the past. Questions about heterosexual relationships also should not to be asked. Lesbian and gay clients may interpret such questions as value judgments about the primacy of heterosexuality (Gartrell, 1984).

Practitioners should also never search for causes of a person's sexual orientation or ask questions about etiology. Seeking answers to these questions implies that nonheterosexual sexual orientations are pathological (Gartrell, 1984). For clients searching for causes, practitioners should acknowledge the importance of this quest to the client but state that there is no certainty about causes.

The Ultimate Goal: Ally/Advocate of LGBT Persons

The highest affirmative level identified by Riddle (1996) is *nurturance*. At this level, practitioners assume that LGBT persons are indispensable to our society. They feel genuine affection and delight about these persons, and they are allies and advocates for them. For heterosexual practitioners who invest in becoming knowledgeable and affirmative, working with LGBT clients can be rewarding. These clients are often high functioning, motivated, and often make more progress than other clients. Generally, they are trying to manage stress or developmental issues instead of trying to cope with psychopathology (Liddle, 1999). If no LGBT practitioners are available in the local area, heterosexual practitioners who are affirmative should make themselves known. If they want potential LGBT clients, they can offer support groups or workshops for LGBT persons, advertise in LGBT newspapers or directories, or let local professionals know they offer affirmative services (Liddle, 1997).

SUMMARY

"Homosexuality" was designated a mental illness by the American Psychiatric Association until 1973 when it was removed from the *Diagnostic and Statistical Manual of Mental Disorders.* The work of Evelyn Hooker that showed that gay men were not mentally ill, and many other research studies that affirmed this about both lesbian and gay persons, helped make this removal possible. All remaining references to "homosexuality" were gone by 1987. Transgender persons are still fighting to get their diagnostic categories removed. Professional organizations representing human services professionals now declare that a same-sex sexual orientation is not a mental illness, but there are still many practitioners and administrators that do not agree with this view. Some practitioners even try to change nonheterosexual sexual orientation although no research supports that this is possible. Other practitioners are affirmative, and lesbian and gay persons report that they like the services they now receive. Being affirmative includes both emotional and intellectual stances as well as language, questions, and the environment. The ultimate goal for an affirmative practitioner is to be an ally/advocate for LGBT persons.

Chapter 8

Overview of Practice Issues with Midlife and Older LGBT Persons

ISSUES LESBIANS MAY EXPERIENCE AT MIDLIFE

Several studies have looked at reasons midlife lesbians seek counseling. Razzano, Matthews, and Hughes (2002) compared the mental health indicators and services utilization factors in a community sample of sixty-three lesbians and a matched sample of fifty-seven heterosexual women. The average age was forty years old. The sample was diverse: 37 percent Caucasian, 28 percent African American, 25 percent Latino (Mexican, Puerto Rican, or Cuban), 7 percent Asian/Pacific Islander, and 3 percent American Indian. More than half (57 percent) were currently married or in a committed relationship. Most had some post–high school education (5 percent with some college or a bachelor's degree); 15 percent a high school education or less. Almost one-third (29 percent) had graduate or professional degrees. Nearly two-thirds were working full time (58 percent), working part time 17 percent, 9 percent unemployed but looking for work. Some (10 percent) were retired or not working due to disability; 5 percent were not currently looking for work. The midlife lesbians reported more use of services in the past five years. There was no significant difference regarding inability to obtain mental health services in the past five years, but a higher proportion of midlife lesbians than heterosexual women reported unmet needs for services from Alcoholics Anonymous (AA) or Narcotics Anonymous (NA) (13 versus 2 percent, significant), and other mental health services (18 versus 4 percent, significant). Significantly more midlife lesbians reported past use of mental health and alcohol and drug-related services, indicating that they were more likely to have sought treatment than heterosexual women. Significantly more midlife lesbians reported past use of antidepressant medications (38 versus 19 percent). A markedly higher proportion of this group reported feelings of depression and issues related to sexual orientation as reasons for seeking mental health services. It was not clear if midlife lesbians are more likely to seek mental health services or genuinely do have higher rates of mental health difficulties. Also, the stress of being a lesbian in a heterosexist society, rather than a lesbian sexual identity itself, may have a stronger influence on the services utilization pattern of midlife lesbians. There was no significant difference between this group and heterosexual women in the history of child sexual experience, history of physical abuse, or current use of antidepressant medications. No significant differences occurred between the two groups of women for nervousness or anxiety, sexual problems, anger, problems sleeping, memory problems, problems with alcohol and or drugs, school and or behavior problems of children, relationship concerns, or other problems as reasons for using mental health services.

The midlife lesbians surveyed by Bradford and Ryan (1991) often sought mental health services mostly for emotional distress and difficulties with lovers. These concerns topped the list of reasons these women gave for seeking a practitioner: feeling sad or depressed (62 percent), difficulties with lovers (62 percent), difficulties with family members (39 percent), feeling anxious or afraid (36 percent), personal growth (32 percent), difficulties with sexual orientation (27 percent), loneliness (24 percent), alcohol and drug difficulties (20 percent), work difficulties (20 percent), difficulties with friends (10 percent), and difficulties with racism (4 percent). Suicide was attempted by 16 percent, most frequently through drug overdose. In this survey, the distress associated with disclosure was significantly associated with long-term use of mental health counseling. No similar surveys have been done with gay persons.

Except for issues of sexual orientation and disclosure, many of the concerns listed can be addressed by standard interventions, including cognitive restructuring, behavioral techniques, self-nurturing, and social-skills training.

Financial Planning

Some midlife lesbians experience worries and anxieties about finances (Bradford & Ryan, 1991). For these clients, referrals to financial planners can be useful as is retirement planning for the many midlife lesbians who are self-supporting (Sang, 1992a, 1992b). Once-married lesbians may need services related to financial security similar to what newly divorced women may need (Bridges & Croteau, 1994).

The characteristics of retirement planning were studied by Mock (2001) in a sample of: thirty-two women in same sex-gender relationships and seven men in same sex-gender relationships, thirty men and women in cohabiting heterosexual relationships, and thirty married heterosexual men and women. All the couples shared many characteristics in their patterns of retirement planning. They planned to retire at similar ages, begin the planning process at similar times, and planned for health care and housing needs to a similar degree. However, married couples have a higher self-rating of post-retirement planning than other couples, to a degree approaching significance. Lesbian couples had a mean self-rating of degree of financial preparation lower than the other three groups, and significantly lower than the married couples.

Planning Ahead

Although financial concerns were the source of most worry for the midlife lesbians studied by Bradford and Ryan (1991), they sought mental health services for emotional distress and relationship problems. If counseling were sought prior to midlife, it was most likely for these same reasons (Sang, 1992a, 1992b). Perhaps this is why they make financial planning a lower priority. The need for advanced planning for successful aging is important, just as it is for all midlife and older persons. In particular, it is imperative that coupled, or single lesbian and gay persons plan ahead for their later years. Planning for older age includes finances, disability and health insurance, and knowledge of the health care and legal systems before a crisis occurs. As noted in Chapter 10, legal documents such as a will and a power of attorney are significant instruments if a partner becomes severely ill or dies (Dunker, 1987; D. Martin & Lyon, 1992). Most of these documents can be used for the protection of single persons as well. LGBT persons must make sure their legal and financial plans are exactly as they wish. Professional advisors, sensitive to their needs, are crucial to prevent troublesome financial and legal issues arising later (R. Jacobson & Wright, 1992; Reid, 1995). Lamda Legal offers resources to help lesbian and gay persons prepare living wills, power-of-attorney forms, and health care proxies (Edwards, 2001).

Social Supports

Although there are many activities and institutions now available, particularly in urban lesbian and gay communities, not all midlife and older lesbians take advantage of these opportunities. Studies of midlife and older lesbians (Adelman, 1988; Kehoe, 1986; Raphael & Robinson, 1984) indicated that only about half of the samples associated themselves with a lesbian and gay organization. Isolation can result from such factors as geographical location or personality factors such as shyness. Other reasons included being closeted, wanting to be with individuals one's own age instead of the usually younger participants in these organizations, or not being a joiner (Sang, 1992a, 1992b). It is important to determine the reasons for low social support and look for modifications.

ISSUES GAY MEN MAY EXPERIENCE
AT MIDLIFE

Midlife Crisis

In midlife, the typical review of one's life can result in a profound shift in identity such as movement from "what I have been and what I am" to "what I will be" (Gurevitch, 2000). For lesbian and gay persons, a midlife review includes not only achievements, strengths, regrets, disappointments, and challenges to self-worth but a review of coming out and the further integration of sexual orientation into their lives (Kimmel & Sang, 1995). The losses and gains normative to midlife are acknowledged but also the acceptance of the fear and limitations imposed by having a stigmatized identity (Glassgold, 1995). This cohort of lesbian and gay persons acknowledge barriers and prejudices they have faced and experience a bittersweet comparison with the relative openness and ease experienced by younger lesbian and gay persons (Gurevitch, 2000).

Both gay and heterosexual men may experience signs associated with a midlife crisis. The classic midlife-crisis signs range from a sense of despair to a sense of renewal and pursuit of youthful ideals (M. Stein, 1983). Kimmel and Sang (1995) indicated that some distresses gay persons may experience during a midlife crisis include

> concerns about issues of mortality and a search for meaning and wholeness in life within a heterosexist society, fear of physical illness, occupation-pertinent stress or not receiving a promotion, family issues including care of aging parents, concerns about one's family lineage, and a feeling that one has lost some masculine prowess with advancing age. (p. 207)

Because they often live on pretense to keep jobs, gay men may also desire more authenticity in their lives. This means no longer presenting as heterosexual but as gay. The death of parents also brings about conscious recognition of or disturbing awareness of one's own finitude (Moss & Moss, 1989).

Many issues that may evoke a crisis for gay persons are similar to the issues that heterosexual persons may also confront (Linde, 1994). These issues can lead to a reassessment for both groups of life decisions, a desire for more purpose and meaning in their lives, and development of a more authentic sense of self (Hopcke, 1992). Frost (1997) recommended the use of groups for midlife gay persons to create more meaning in their lives, to come to love themselves and others, and to contemplate issues of generativity or ways to give back to the lesbian and gay community or to society at large.

Not all life events, or the timing of some events, are the same for heterosexual and gay persons. The shake-up and transformation of a settled life pattern due to a midlife crisis scenario may occur much earlier for many gay persons. The classic midlife-crisis pattern, for example, occurs in the late thirties or early forties. Persons supposedly experience pressures to switch from outward orientation to an inward reflection and experience a transformation. For gay persons, however, this switch may occur during the coming out and disclosure processes which include the distress of coping with heterosexism (Hopcke, 1992). Gay persons may develop competence in dealing with crises early because of the unique experience of heterosexism (Kimmel & Sang, 1995).

Gay persons may also experience a crisis of another kind during midlife. According to Linde (1994), midlife may confront gay persons with a crisis of identity and social interaction. Those who link much of their self-esteem to physical attractiveness and appearance may experience anxiety about losing these attributes. They may feel increasingly repudiated and abandoned. Bennett and Thompson (1990) asked a sample of gay persons what age they thought gay persons perceived as the beginning of middle and old age. They believed that gay persons thought middle age began on average at thirty-nine and old age at fifty-four. These are substantially younger ages than than the ages reported by heterosexuals. L. M. Woolf (2002) pointed out that the youth orientation of the community may account for accelerated aging. However, other studies reported no difference between lesbian and gay persons and heterosexuals in terms of what age they saw as beginning middle age or old age (Dorfman et al., 1995). Accelerated aging seems to be a concern for only a small group of gay persons and of no concern among lesbians (Hostetler, 2000). Linde suggested that the task for gay persons is to redefine their self-worth as well as discover new ways to associate with other persons who do not emulate a youthful version of sexual attractiveness.

HIV/AIDS

One issue that has had a momentous impact on midlife for many gay and bisexual men is HIV/AIDS, which is transmitted mainly through male-to-male unprotected sex. Although lesbian sex has not been a major mode of transmission, lesbians are also at risk if they participate in injection drug use and/or have sex with men (Shankle et al., 2003). Increasing evidence indicates that the rate of HIV infection among transgender women is high. In California, this risk of infection may even surpass that for gay and bisexual men (e.g., Sykes, 1999). Many transgender women participate in risky sexual behaviors as well as share needles during the injection of hormones or drugs (Nemoto, 1999).

Most of the literature on HIV/AIDS focuses on gay persons because of the major impact on the gay community. Since the 1980s, gay men have been confronted with the illness and death of their friends, partners, and many others in their community, and with the fear of their own diagnosis of HIV (Paul et al.,1995).

Some midlife gay persons with HIV are homeless. Meris (2001) studied a small group of aging homeless HIV-infected gay men (over age fifty) (range from fifty-two to seventy-one years, mean age fifty-nine) living in the meat-packing district of New York City. They had diverse ethnic backgrounds: two Caucasians, four African Americans, and one Puerto-Rican American. All had completed high school and two had some college. They all had prior stable careers. At the time of the study, however, they had been homeless for an average of 1.46 years and had been living with the HIV virus from two to fourteen years with an average of 6.82 years. Some had succumbed to substance abuse that resulted in financial ruin and abandonment by family and others. Two of the African-American men left their families in the South to live on the streets in New York City. They occasionally worked part time; three were eligible for governmental assistance but routinely used the money for drugs and alcohol.

The respondents were a street family for one another. They shared nights in subway stations, parks, and street sidewalks, stood in soup lines, weathered through winters and rainy days; and helped one another to emergency rooms for urgent medical care. They preferred the streets to the shelter system of New York City. Deaths wiped out their social support networks both prior to their homeless experiences and on the street. They had all seen family members and friends die from AIDS. They recalled a range of seven to thirty-one AIDS-related deaths, with an average of fifteen deaths. They also witnessed other deaths including those from murder, tuberculosis, lung cancer, prostate cancer, heart attack, pneumonia, gay bashing, and diabetes. The deceased persons were confidants, brothers, and friends. These men were often left to cope with multiple bereavements in isolation. These losses were not addressed by mental health workers, nor were mental health difficulties including acute depression, attention deficit disorders, hallucinations, paranoia, uncontrollable rage, and sabotaged ties with remaining family and social networks. All these men reported periods of depression during their time on the streets but none were ever medically treated for even severe depression. They all lived with various sexually transmitted diseases (STDs) but were never treated for them. Alcoholism and other substance use dominated the participants' existence that they proclaimed were part of the homeless culture. These men need culturally appropriate (gay and homeless-sensitive) outreach services so they can access mental health and grief care systems, and experience a better quality of life.

The deaths from AIDS that the men experienced were just a part of what has happened to the whole midlife cohort of gay men. As a result of this epidemic, the social networks of midlife gay persons hardly exist in some parts of the country. Many survivors will face their later years without the support of friends and lovers who died of this disease (Boxer, 1997; Kimmel & Sang, 1995; Paul et al., 1995). For those living with their own illness and impending death, among the greatest need for most of them is validation and love from others. Some also reported that spirituality and a higher power were their greatest needs (L. B. Brown et al., 2001).

Those infected with the HIV virus are confronted with premature mortality (Berger & Kelly, 2001). This psychological crisis results in an "AIDS-induced midlife" (Hopcke, 1992, p. 108). They face the challenge of being out of time at midlife or off time in terms of normative developmental schedules. Upon learning that they are infected with HIV many are forced to reflect on their lives and make changes for the better long before this desire occurs, usually at the normative time of midlife (Hopcke, 1992). Developmental schedules are collapsed and events that usually come later occur, such as the loss of loved ones and the realization of the finitude of life (Bennett & Thompson, 1990; Borden, 1989; 1992; J. Kelly, 1980).

In addition to the persons with AIDS, this disease also affects those who are involved as caregivers of friends and partners, or others such as volunteers for AIDS service organizations. Some of these persons may seek human services because of anger, loneliness, depression, anxiety, and "survivor's guilt." In addition, AIDS not only interrupts the normal aging process for those with the disease; it can also prematurely age the caregivers (L. B. Brown et al., 2001).

ISSUES THAT OLDER LESBIAN AND GAY PERSONS MAY EXPERIENCE

Older lesbian and gay persons have needs and concerns that are similar to those of older heterosexuals such as health, income, transportation, planning and funding retirement years, isolation, loneliness, bereavement, developing future primary relationships, making new friends, lack of support, housing, jobs and job training, and meaningful use of leisure time. There may also be concerns with body changes, lessening mobility, and being old in a youth-oriented society (Adleman et al., 1993; Kehoe, 1986; Kochman, 1997; Lee, 1987; Lucco, 1987; McDougall, 1993; Quam & Whitford, 1992).

What is different is that older lesbian and gay persons must contend with the effects of heterosexism such as myths and stereotypes, lack of recognition, and heterosexist policies especially in the health care system (Tully, 2000). Several issues that may bring older lesbian and gay persons to a practitioner are discussed here along with practice principles and the usefulness of group services.

HIV/AIDS

Most (93 percent) older lesbian and gay persons studied by Grossman et al. (2001) knew persons diagnosed with HIV/AIDS, and 90 percent knew someone who died from HIV/AIDS. Almost half (47 percent) reported that they knew three or more people who had died from HIV/AIDS. In a study of sixty-nine gay persons ages thirty-six to seventy-nine (most fifty to sixty-five), L. B. Brown et al. (2001) found that they felt HIV/AIDS had a devastating effect on older gay men. However, because this older generation was less involved in the gay sexual culture at the time of mass infection, relatively few of them contracted HIV (Boxer, 1997). Most of the older gay persons (90 percent) in Grossman et al.'s sample reported that they were very unlikely or unlikely to become infected with HIV, 6 percent did not know, 2 percent likely or very likely to be infected, and 2 percent infected. Of the 2 percent who reported they were HIV infected, eight were men and one a woman. The low HIV rates for older gay persons does not mean they are not at risk. Also, early HIV symptoms such as weight loss, fatigue, decreased mental and physical abilities, can be mistaken for other diseases such as Alzheimer's, Parkinson's, and respiratory disease (Williams & Donnelly, 2002).

Some gay persons who were infected at an earlier age are now living into their older years. Many of those who fell ill during the 1980s were gay persons in their thirties and forties. Those who survived are now in their forties, fifties, and sixties. These men face the multiple challenges of growing older and coping with chronic illness (Berger & Kelly, 2001). Older gay and bisexual men with HIV have more symptoms and illnesses than younger persons. HIV may also elevate the risk of cancers, cognitive impairment, and mortality. Older persons may also have more difficulty in metabolizing drugs to treat HIV/AIDS (Shankle et al., 2003). Older LGBT persons may often bear substantial caretaking responsibility due to HIV/AIDS among their peers or even younger friends (Williams & Donnelly, 2002).

Older gay and bisexual men can benefit from primary prevention efforts. AIDS prevention education, however, has been almost exclusively focused on young and middle-aged populations (Feldman, 1994). Only in the gay community have prevention campaigns targeted all age groups. Sexual practices among older gay and bisexual men are generally similar to younger gay and bisexual men although they are less likely to have anal intercourse with causal partners (Ven et al., 1997). Data collected from gay persons age fifty or older show that these campaigns can help reduce risk behaviors in this population once they are aware of how to avoid infection (Stall & Catania, 1994). The most important way to do this is to never have unprotected sex with another male. The other male could be infected. Male-to-male unprotected sex with an infected partner accounts for 60 percent of all HIV infection (Linsk, 1997; Stall & Catania, 1994).

In general, the prevalence of AIDS is thought to have leveled off among older gay men in large cities (Vincke, Bolton, and Miller, 1997). However, those who have HIV/AIDS often feel marginalized by the services available to them (Williams & Donnelly, 2002).

Dealing with Internalized Oppression and Ageism

Most older lesbian and gay persons studied by Grossman et al. (2001) reported low levels of internalized oppression, but men reported significantly more negative attitudes toward same sex-gender sexual orientation than women. Those living alone reported more internalized oppression than those living with a partner. No differences were found in sexual orientation. The older one was, the more likely a person was to report internalized oppression. Contact with more people appears to also be related. Those who were members of and who had greater levels of involvement with lesbian or gay organizations had less internalized oppression. Individuals with more people in their support networks also reported less internalized oppression. Victmization was not related.

Aside from contact with others and greater involvement in organizations, recommendations for dealing with ageism also apply to dealing with internalized oppression. As LGB persons age they may need assistance in overcoming negative attitudes about aging. This requires accomplishing several tasks, such as seeking out positive role models for successful aging, developing new age-suitable standards of attractiveness, visualizing a positive future as mature adults, and working on life planning and goal setting. Diverse models of older lesbian and gay persons can counter stereotypical and stigmatized images and provide alternative ways to approach older age (Kooden, 1997). The most useful models are older lesbian and gay persons who are active, productive, self-motivated, and sexual (Friend, 1990). Interactions with lesbian and gay persons of different ages can also provide varied role models as well as social stimulation (Friend, 1987). Affirmative books with accurate information countering myths and misconceptions of older lesbian and gay persons can also help (Friend, 1987). Several possibilities include *Gay and Gray* by Berger (1996) and *Rubyfruit Jungle* by R. Brown (1973).

Groups such as Old Lesbians Organizing for Change (OLOC, <http://www.oloc.org>), Senior Action in a Gay Environment (SAGE, http://www.sageusa.org>), and Pride Senior Network (PSN, <http://www.pridesenior.org/index.htm>) have addressed ageism in the GLBT community. They call for LGBT persons to examine their own ageism and take action to remedy the ageism of the LGBT communities. Individuals need to eliminate ageist stereotypes and language, listen to and consider older persons as serious, involve them in decision-making and policy bodies, provide opportunities for intergenerational personal and social interaction, and take on the political issues that concern older persons such as health care and economic security issues (Cahill et al., 2000).

Housing

With aging, potential loss of income and concern over independent and supportive living arrangement heightens. This concern may be exacerbated by loss of a life partner or diminishment of support groups due to disability, chronic illness, or death. A few corporations, institutions, agencies, and municipalities now provide domestic partners with health and retirement benefits. However, the vast majority of older lesbian and gay persons do not have such options available. Without careful financial and estate planning, the surviving partner may be forced out of his or her home or face other income-related housing problems (Claes & Moore, 2000). Surviving partners may not only be evicted from the homes they have lived in for many years, but see treasures collected during their partnerships leave with relatives (Wojciechowski, 1998). Even if couples are financially secure and have planned ahead by investigating housing options, such as life-care communities or assisted-living facilities, they may find they are not allowed to live together or their application is suddenly withdrawn if their relationship is disclosed (Claes & Moore, 2000).

Lesbian and gay baby boomers who have been out most of their adult lives will increasingly refuse to hide their identities in any housing option. They will want to live with their lifetime partners or have visitation privileges. These concerns have led to calls for the development of long-term care facilities and retirement communities specifically designed and marketed for lesbian and gay residents. Those now in their seventies and eighties might not want to live in a place called Rainbow Gardens. However, as one becomes frail and life more difficult, a place that is affirming, comfortable, and safe is of the utmost importance (Edwards, 2001).

Lucco (1987) did a preliminary study to gauge interest among older lesbians and gay persons for planned retirement housing. The sample included 399 gay persons and fifty-seven lesbians with an average age of sixty-three. Most lived alone, were still working, and had a higher socioeconomic status than the general older population. Lucco pointed out that older lesbians and gay persons anticipated entry in a retirement community at a considerably lower age than the average age of seventy-five.

A large majority of Lucco's (1987) respondents (87.7 percent) were interested in planned retirement housing that focused on the needs of lesbian and gay persons and supported a range of services. Security and health services were the most desired. Many respondents were willing to move long distances to live in such housing.

Two-thirds (63 percent) of lesbians and 45 percent of the gay persons in Almvig's (1982) sample indicated they would join a lesbian and gay retirement village. Most lesbians in Kehoe's (1986) study indicated preference for exclusively lesbian or lesbian and gay retirement centers and nursing homes. Sixty percent of Robinson's (1980) study of twenty lesbians ages fifty and older were positive about a lesbian, women's, or lesbian and gay retirement community. None expressed interest in a community that included heterosexuals. Almost two-thirds (62 percent) of Quam and Whitford's (1992) sample was willing to consider living in a lesbian only or gay only retirement community or in one with both sex-genders. Fewer (44 percent) respondents would consider a general population community. Lesbians (53.8 percent) expressed more interest in a community for women only than gay persons (24.4 percent) in a community for men only. Most lesbians (79.5 percent) preferred a lesbian only community. The American Association of Homes and Services for the Aging (AAHSA) now includes sessions at annual conferences on lesbian and gay issues in terms of housing (Connolly, 1996).

The New York Community Trust, a city grants organization, awarded the New York City–based SAGE organization money to study the feasibility of building a lesbian- and gay-oriented retirement home (Mann, 1997). The survey done by SAGE found that half of the older LGBT persons in New York City desired to lower their cost of living as a major reason for moving into special-needs housing. Most cited failing health and the need for assistance as the reason to move to such housing. Half said they would move to avoid having to live alone. More than two-thirds (65 percent) were currently living alone. A survey of GLBT senior service and housing advocates in San Francisco found that the vast majority wanted to live in a LGBT housing development (Hamburger, 1997).

Several housing projects for lesbian and gay persons across the country are in various stages of development. This includes projects underway for SAGE and the Gay and Lesbian Association of Retiring Persons (GLARP) in Palm Springs, California, for both lesbian and gay persons (Shankle et al., 2003). The Queen City Community Development corporation is building a multigenerational, multipurpose facility that will house the Seattle Gay Cultural Center and a Senior Housing Project in Seattle, Washington. Our Town is planning a facility near San Francisco, as is Metropolitan Community Homes, a project of the Metropolitan Community Church. A project called Stonewall Communities is planning a housing development in the middle of Boston for lesbian and gay persons. Established in 1988, Rainbow Gardens (1999) of Durango, Colorado, is seeking to build retirement and assisted-living centers throughout the United States that are friendly to lesbian and gay persons (Cahill et al., 2000). RainbowVision Properties in Northern New Mexico has proposed 100 independent and thirty-five assisted-living units. This organization is negotiating a downtown property purchase. Birds of a Feather, near Pecos, New Mexico, has 140 acres with a twenty-three-home clustered subdivision primarily for lesbians. A San Francisco non-profit housing group, Rainbow Adult Community Housing, now known as Open House, is seeking to build the first mixed-income housing unit for older LGBT persons. The group received $250,000 from state government sources to perform feasibility studies on the project. It will house 330 persons and will include a mixture of market-rate and subsidized apartments aimed at lower- and middle-income older LGBT persons. There will be a theater, café, fitness center, and a dementia and Alzheimer's disease care unit (Quittner, 2002). Open House is a retirement housing development in the planning stages in San Francisco, and GL Eldercare will be located in Los Angeles. Housing projects now open include: the Palms in Manasota in Palmetto, Florida, and the Resort on Carefree Boulevard in Fort Myers, Florida, which is a private, gated independent community with one- to three-bedroom homes sold at market value (Cahill et al., 2000). The Hollywood Retirement Complex is expected to open in 2005 (Lelyveld, 2003). Other housing developments include: Gay Family Compound in Guerneville, California, and Rainbow Manor in Ottawa, Canada (Chernin & Johnson, 2003). The Lesbian and Gay Aging Issues Network (LGAIN) includes an extensive list of housing developments and updates on progress (American Society on Aging, 2004).

Although these are useful developments, there are not enough retirement, assisted-living, and life-care facilities to meet the growing need of this older population overall. There are no large-scale corporate initiatives to develop them (Claes & W. R. Moore, 2000). In addition, any of the existing or proposed long-term care models are expensive, and since most LGBT older persons depend only on Social Security, Medicare, and/or Medicaid, they are unlikely to be able to afford any of them (Shankle et al., 2003). Without some type of subsidy, lower socioeconomic status (SES) LGBT persons will have difficulty finding suitable housing (Baron & Cramer, 2000).

End-of-Life Issues

Long-Term Care Facilities

Older lesbian and gay persons fear dying in a nursing home or other long-term care facility without family or friends (Berger, 1996; L. B. Brown et al., 2001; Kehoe, 1989; Lieberman & Tobin, 1983).

Almost everything in nursing homes is heterosexually focused or biased, from a male resident talking about his wife and children, pictures on the walls showing only heterosexual couples, and a staff not trained to work with LGBT persons. This kind of environment can result in an LGB or T resident feeling isolated, unacknowledged, and depressed (Edwards, 2001).

It was suggested by Fullmer et al. (1999) that a manual be developed that explains current knowledge about older lesbian and gay persons, cases studies, and ways to reach out to this population. There should be an emphasis on empowerment of these clients with the use of groups to provide a venue for telling life stories and exploring shared experiences, concerns, and effective strategies for personal success. A director of policy and education of Senior Action in a Gay Environment (SAGE) suggested that in facilities for older lesbian and gay persons, pictures should be hung of same sex-gender couples together or a group of these couples in a park setting. These facilities should provide private rooms for lesbian and gay couples if they are provided for heterosexual couples. Gay pride activities need to be events celebrated in the facilities (Edwards, 2001).

End-of-Life Care

Perspectives on end-of-life care were sought from 575 participants recruited by Stein and Bonuck (2001) through community-based health care and social service organizations serving the lesbian and gay community primarily in the New York City metropolitan area. The sample included women (36 percent) and men (63 percent) of various ages and racial/ethnic and religious/spiritual backgrounds. Also, 10 percent were HIV positive. The perspectives of this sample on end-of-life care were generally consistent with findings from other attitudinal studies on this topic. A majority supported legalizing physician-assisted suicide (PAS) and preferred a palliative approach to end-of-life care even if it shortened life. Combining support for legalizing PAS under both broad and narrow situations, 92 percent of lesbian and gay persons endorsed legalization versus 65 percent among adults nationwide. The gay participants reported the strongest support for PAS and palliative care (83 percent). African Americans were much less likely to endorse efforts to legalize assisted suicide than whites and Latinos, although they were willing to consider it for themselves. Jewish respondents were more favorable to legalization of PAS under a wide variety of circumstances than were Catholic or Protestant peers. Here again, despite religion, they were willing to consider PAS for themselves and they preferred palliative approaches to end-of-life care for themselves. Older respondents were more likely to support PAS as a policy or personal matter. Most (93 percent) respondents over age sixty supported the legalization of PAS and 80 percent could imagine requesting it for themselves.

The sample studied by G. L. Stein and Bonuck (2001) had a high degree of knowledge about living wills (90 percent) and health care proxies (72 percent). The high level of awareness about advance directives probably reflect their connections to social service and health care organizations serving lesbian and gay communities. On the other hand, less than half completed advance directives of a health care proxy (42 percent) or living will (38 percent). Yet compared to adults generally (28 percent), they signed advance directives at a much higher rate. Health care proxies are critical for lesbian and gay persons who want partners or friends to make medical decisions for them in times of incapacity. Yet among the 43 percent who wished to have their partner make medical decisions, only half had actually named these persons in an advance directive.

PRACTICE PRINCIPLES FOR WORKING WITH OLDER LESBIAN AND GAY PERSONS

A set of practice principles for working with older lesbian and gay persons, developed by Humphreys and Quam (1998), addresses attitudes, knowledge, and skills. These principles, which could also apply to midlife lesbian and gay persons, include the following:

- *Respect these persons' right to privacy and confidentiality.* Many older lesbian and gay persons do not want their sexual orientation known.
- *Recognize diversity among older LGB persons.* Some are partnered, some have children, and some are single. The age at which they discovered they were gay, lesbian, or bisexual could have been at twenty, fifty, or later. Different persons are at different levels of comfort with their sexual orientation and in how open or closeted they are. Some are out to everyone whereas

others might never have acknowledged their sexual identity to anyone. Some might have a history of acceptance from family and friends whereas others might have experienced humiliating discrimination and rejection. Important differences also emerge depending on the era in which they were born and when they acknowledged a lesbian, gay, or bisexual orientation. S. Jacobson (1995) pointed out that both midlife and older lesbian and gay persons might use different terminology to refer to themselves and their sexual orientation than younger lesbian and gay persons do. As noted ealier in this book, it is important to inquire about and use terms that are most comfortable for the client. In addition, although a sexual history might appear as if the client is bisexual, the client, if an older person, might not use this term.

- *Recognize that not all the difficulties experienced by a person are associated with being old or gay, lesbian, or bisexual.* It is easy to fall into an ageist trap of thinking that because someone is old, he or she is tired or frail. Similarly, a heterosexist bias might lead the practitioner to see clients as frightened or depressed when clients can feel this way about many things other than age or sexual orientation.

- *Treat identified family as family.* As discussed in various places in this book, lesbian and gay persons create their own families. Older lesbian and gay persons fear that in times of critical decisions about their health, members of their family of choice will not be acknowledged as the persons the client wants involved in the decisions.

- *Plan activities and discussions that are neutral with respect to sexual orientation.* Instead of a Valentine's Day discussion about "husbands and wives," the topic can be "those I have loved." Instead of dances for male and female partners, have round dances and ethnic dancing that do not have this requirement.

- *Create a staff atmosphere that is open to discussion about differences among clients and an environment that does not tolerate discrimination based on sexual identity or gender expression.* Although many agencies do good work with staff training and developing sensitivity to diversity, including sexual identity and gender expression, personnel changes over time. New questions arise particularly with new clients and circumstances that might challenge the norms of an agency. The environment needs to be one in which staff members can safely express their lack of knowledge about these challenges or how to handle them.

SUMMARY

Except for issues concerning sexual orientation and disclosure, many concerns that lesbian and gay persons bring to a social services practitioner can be addressed by standard interventions such as cognitive restructuring, behavioral techniques, self-nurturing, and social skills training. Other issues that may need to be addressed include financial planning and planning for one's older years, such as knowing where to get affirmative medical care, obtaining social supports, and balancing roles. In addition, gay persons may be dealing with a midlife crisis, HIV/AIDS, or both. Everyone may be dealing with internalized ageism and oppression. Housing may be another concern, especially for older lesbian and gay persons. Other concerns may be long-term care facilities and end-of-life care.

Chapter 9

Practice with Coming-Out and Disclosure Issues

COMING-OUT ISSUES FOR LESBIAN AND GAY PERSONS

Although variability exists among midlife and older lesbians and gay persons, they have common experiences coping with heterosexism and with coming out and making disclosures. Although coming out is now happening at younger ages, it can happen at any age (Charbonneau & Lander, 1991; Sang, 1992). Professional help might be sought because of new feelings about someone of the same sex-gender, or these feelings may be discovered during counseling. LGB individuals may need assistance in conceptualizing coming out as a life transition which can be stressful and painful. Clarifying what challenges they may experience can facilitate a more positive transition (Bridges & Croteau, 1994).

Early in the Process

The main task for affirmative practitioners is to assist clients in exploring and discovering whatever self-identification they feel is "their own." Until and unless clients are ready to self-identify with a label, it is important not to mention one or assign a category to them. The practitioner can encourage clients who feel confused about their sexual identity or are just beginning to explore a nonheterosexual identity to discover their own needs and desires without pressure or censorship (Matteson, 1996a). One can express to confused clients that it is all right to declare that they are gay, lesbian, or bisexual, or heterosexual; to feel confused; to go back and forth; and to change their minds. Accept clients as they are, no matter where this process takes them (Drescher, 1998; Mallon, 1998a).

Although many practitioners may be familiar with the Kinsey scale that categorizes sexual orientation—from "heterosexual" to "homosexual"—they may not be familiar with the many revisions of it (Kinsey et al., 1948; Kinsey et al., 1953). Even though none of the existing scales are yet satisfactory, some of the multidimensional scales such as the Klein Sexual Orientation Grid (Klein et al., 1985) can be useful in assisting clients who feel confused about their sexual identity. Practice can focus on the various aspects of their attraction to men and to women, including sexual behavior, fantasy, and emotional or affectional intimacy. If clients use categorical labels such as bisexual or gay, practitioners can help them explore what these labels mean to them (Stokes, Miller, & Mundhenk, 1998).

Sequential identity-development models can provide clues of what to look for in a client's identity development, aid a client in understanding possible pathways to identity development, normalize a client's feelings and experiences, provide tasks for a client to anticipate, and suggest interventions. However, the can also represent the way in which only some persons experience the coming-out process, obscure or invalidate issues unique to some persons, and usually imply a stable resolution to identification when one reaches the final stages (Bohan, 1996; Rust, 1996a). It is best to inquire what the client's actual experiences are because they may vary from the established coming-out models. Clients will also fluctuate in the timing of moving from the initial discovery of same sex-gender sexual orientation through other stages. Many variables in one's social context will affect the coming-out process and the timing of the various stages, or even stopping and not going further. The practitioner's task is not to help clients arrive at a firm and fixed identity, nor to speed it along, but instead to support flexibility in exploring sexual identity.

Another complication regarding identity-development models is that LGB identities are not fixed categories (Cass, 1996). Nor are they limited to two categories: heterosexual and "homosexual." Persons may experience sexual feelings for both women and men. This may be a transitional state or more representative of bisexuality. As discussed in Chapter 1, sexual identification is so complex that trying to fit oneself into a narrow and confining identity may not match what is more authentic for a particular person. Some clients also experience genuine fluidity among identities. Women's sexual identity may especially be fluid and more defined by particular relationships or social settings (Rust, 1993; Savin-Williams & Diamond, 1999). This suggests the need for adopting a constructionist stance as well as the essentialist stance (Bohan, 1996). Many clients believe their sexual identity is internal to them and this should be respected.

Several other issues that may arise for clients at early stages of coming out were identified by Levy (1995), including validation of a new self-concept resulting from the changes in self-concept during coming out, and challenging negative thoughts about themselves if internalized oppression surfaces. Because of the many difficult issues clients confront at this stage, supportive groups and educational approaches can be useful (Guidry, 1999).

If not already experienced, persons coming out will eventually want to meet and interact with other LGB persons. This can be facilitated in local support groups (Degges-White, Rice, & Myers, 2000). Or, they can be directed to community centers, bookstores, special-interest groups, and a variety of other places where LGB persons congregate. There are also LGB newspapers and phone books (listed under gay or lambda) that list LGB organizations and activities (Rust, 1996a).

Issues for Persons from Prior Marriages

If prior self-identification included heterosexual marriage, making the shift to a positive self-identification as lesbian may be difficult, as found in 53 percent of Wyers' (1987) sample of formerly married lesbians. There may be difficulties such as "loss of economic support, fear of loss of support from family and friends, getting adjusted to another culture with its own customs, and possibly a limited opportunity to meet other lesbians of their age" (Sang, 1992a, pp. 39-40). According to Bridges and Croteau (1994), it is important to provide these women accurate and affirming views of lesbians to counter previous negative images. The primary means for this are positive contacts with other lesbians along with affirmative books, support groups, and cognitive restructuring.

When older gay persons studied by Herdt et al. (1997) had been in long-term marriages and had little or no experience with the gay community, they often struggled with tasks usually associated with adolescence instead of with midlife. They were suddenly in an unfamiliar world and experienced considerable uncertainty. Not only did they have to redefine themselves, but they also had to figure out how to fit in a new environment. Some felt that heterosexual marriage did not prepare them for being single and dating in this new world. They expressed a sense of "being different" from other gay persons because of their many years in a heterosexual marriage. They wondered whether gay persons not formerly married could understand the significance of their children to them, how time-consuming children can be, the difficulties regarding divorce, the difficulties of coming out in later life, and the difficulties of disclosure to their children. The differences left them feeling as if they were living in two worlds. These persons and lesbians with similar experiences may present different issues in counseling than those with a different history. Some of them may want to learn dating skills to use in the lesbian and gay communities and want support groups for persons in situations such as theirs.

COMING-OUT ISSUES FOR BISEXUAL PERSONS

Bisexual clients may seek assistance for and express both identity concerns (how to handle difficulties and complications of adopting a bisexual identity) and system concerns (how to handle multiple relationships if desired and how to find supports for bisexual relationships). These and additional issues, identified by Matteson (1996b) and others, are listed here:

1. *Personal and social risk taking:* Is the client willing to take personal and social risks? Personal risks include both psychological risks such as internalized oppression and physical risks such as HIV/AIDS and harassment or bashing. An example of a social risk is being fired from a job.
2. *Link between sex and intimacy:* Are sex and intimacy viewed as occurring together or as separate processes? Are they associated with one or both sex-genders? How significant is each of these factors to clients? Are clients open to recreational sex?
3. *Importance of the sex-gender of a partner:* Are one's attractions more for women or men? Or is the sex-gender of a partner not a significant determinant of partner choice?

4. *Desire for monogamous relationships or concurrent partners:* Is monogamy preferred or does the client seek more than one partner?

5. *Ambiguity, confusion, and complexity:* Can the client tolerate these experiences that accompany their relationships? Conclusions about this can be sorted out by fantasy for some clients whereas for others real-life experience is necessary. Confusion about sexual orientation is especially intense during the early stages of bisexual identity development. Confusion may lead some persons with attractions to both sex-genders to self-identify as lesbian or gay or as heterosexual. Practitioners can help these clients reframe their confusion as a response to society's heterosexism and to simplistic dichotomous views of sexuality (Stokes & Damon, 1995).

6. *Lack of social confirmation for bisexual experience:* Because of the stereotypes and myths associated with bisexual persons, they may have trouble attaining social validation from heterosexual and gay and lesbian persons. Practitioners can facilitate comfort with bisexual attractions by affirming that attraction to persons of both sex-genders is legitimate and acceptable. This may be the only "therapy" many clients need (Fox, 1991; Stokes & Damon, 1995).

7. *Overcoming self-oppression:* Bisexual persons struggle with heterosexism because of their attractions to persons of their own sex-gender. They are also at odds with taboos about extramarital sex or multiple relationships (Matteson, 1996b). It is important for them to become acquainted with persons who are comfortable with their bisexual orientation. Coming-out groups and affirmative readings can be helpful (Lourea, 1985; Paul, 1988). Autobiographical accounts of what other bisexual men and women experienced in coming out and how they successfully moved through the process can help. Examples are in the Off Pink Collective (1988).

8. *Guilt:* If clients who are exploring coming out as bisexual are presently in a committed heterosexual link, they may feel guilty if they break the expectation of sexual exclusivity. Support networks can help these persons and their partners to cope with this situation (Matteson, 1995).

9. *Grief:* Whether gay, lesbian, or bisexual, coming out often involves grief (for example, Barron, 1996; C. A. Thompson, 1992), as persons recognize that dreams and desires they pursued earlier no longer work for them. These dreams and desires might have included monogamy and a traditional life of heterosexual marriage with children. These persons may also grieve the loss of support from some heterosexual friends and relatives.

10. *Finding support networks:* It is essential for bisexual clients to interact with positive models of bisexual identity. If clients are unaware of resources, practitioners can help them identify places where they can meet others with the same sexual orientation and common interests. These contacts can help clients sort out the direction of their sexual feelings and behaviors (Matteson, 1996b).

COMING-OUT ISSUES FOR TRANSGENDER PERSONS

Transgender persons may seek a practitioner because of the need to understand a compulsive desire to cross-dress; the belief that they are different from others or perverted, mentally ill, or sinful; the belief that they are in the wrong body; and the strong dislike of their genitals. Other common issues in the transgender client population include shame, depression, guilt, low self-esteem, low sense of competence, social isolation, substance misuse, and suicidal behaviors. They are also dealing with secretiveness regarding feelings about being in the wrong body (Anderson, 1998). An extensive list of assessment factors for use with transgender persons—including those related to health history, mental health history, legal history, sexual history, sex-gender continuum placement—is provided by Cole et al. (2000).

As practitioners, we must communicate to transgender clients that whatever they present about themselves is totally acceptable. We must communicate that we value and appreciate diversity. Anderson (1998) noted that another major task for the practitioner is to provide accurate and meaningful information for transgender clients. Support groups are particularly helpful for transgender persons to test out their identities. In support groups, transgender persons studied by

Gagné et al. felt full acceptance and freedom to be themselves for the first time. If others in these groups accepted them, they often felt that they were truly transgender. Organizations, publications, and online services that focus on transgender persons are also helpful.

Another concern for transgender clients, if they decide to pursue this course, is sexual reassignment surgery (SRS). If clients are thinking about SRS but do not know much about it, they need information about requirements on becoming candidates for the surgery and where to obtain resources to meet other needs such as electrolysis, hormonal intervention, and cosmetic surgery. Reality testing and examination of future expectations are also important (Anderson, 1998).

Centers should be recommended that do not coerce clients into specific outcomes or exclude persons deemed too young, too old, or who will not "pass" well in the new sex-gender. These centers also should not require clients to cross-live full-time as a condition for initiating hormone therapy. This requirement creates a dangerous potential for hate crimes because prior to hormone treatment, these persons can be easily noticed. Only a few such centers exist in the United States: the University of Michigan Comprehensive Gender Services Program and the University of Minnesota Program in Human Sexuality (Cole et al., 2000).

Work with these clients usually takes a minimum of six months before surgery and then some time following surgery. Some transgender persons have no preparation for the period following SRS and do not know the locations of needed services. Others who relocate to "start a new life" may feel isolated and lonely. The practitioner can be most helpful in a supportive role, bolstering coping skills and furnishing information about community services. These clients also need assistance in coping with discrimination and victimization. They need an accurate assessment of how well they pass as the new gender and must prepare to cope if identified by others as transgender, if this matters to them. Practitioners can address needed modifications in appearance and behavior. They may also need to address relationship stress or specific transition periods such as when children mature or when partners enter or leave their lives (Anderson, 1998).

Persons who want SRS but cannot obtain it because of health or financial reasons may also require considerable support. They must come to terms with their unfulfilled dreams of matching their bodies with their sex-gender. Practitioners can help them to cross-live successfully without surgical modification of their bodies. The primary goals with all transgender clients are experiencing relief of painful feelings and self-assessments, making informed decisions, and living productive and fulfilling lives (Anderson, 1998).

DISCLOSURES

Clients must decide what to do about disclosures. Practitioners should never impose personal views about this issue on clients—with one exception. When clients are HIV positive or have AIDS and have not disclosed this information to their partners, practitioners must insist that clients make this information known (Shernoff, 1998).

If clients determine that there may be benefits from disclosures, practitioners can help them assess these situations (Browning et al. 1991). Can they handle the repercussions of disclosing a gay, lesbian, or bisexual identity in their interpersonal lives? One way to assess this is to ask clients to envision the reactions of others to disclosures. How would their mother/father, best friend, girlfriend/ boyfriend, wife/husband, children, religious leader/employer react and how would clients respond? Which friends would be supportive? If married, what would be the implications for marriage and how would they feel about that? (Rust, 1996a).

If clients are committed to disclosures, they can be helped to make thoughtful choices about whom, when, where, and how (Williamson, 1998). *Who* involves which persons to tell. Clients have an uncanny ability to predict responses to startling information and have a sense of which persons are most likely to be supportive (Kuehlwein, 1992). This helps them anticipate the best and worst situations (Williamson, 1998). Based on this kind of information, it is useful to develop a ranked sequence of persons they want to tell. Because it often takes weeks or months to work through feelings about a particular disclosure, it is best not to disclose to everyone simultaneously (Gartrell, 1984).

When involves timing and the issue of when one should not disclose (Williamson, 1998). Clients should make disclosures when they are feeling positive about themselves rather than when they are feeling vulnerable. They should feel prepared instead of making impulsive or reactive disclosures (Gartrell, 1984).

Where involves variations such as one person at a time or in a group and what type of group. *How* involves the style of disclosure such as a subtle statement, a strong statement, or a matter-of-fact statement (Williamson, 1998). The strongest or the most forward type of disclosure is the "Queer Nation" approach in which persons announce their sexual orientation publicly by every act they do, with the accompanying attitude that it is unimportant whether others like them or not (Esterberg, 1996; Klein, 1993). Most persons are subtler than this even in matter-of-fact disclosures, such as when a woman says she dated a woman last weekend (Pope, 1995).

In terms of the *how,* or the methods for making disclosures, what "disclosure skills" do clients have? Are they up to the task, or do they need further coaching and time to prepare (Williamson, 1998)? If clients need coaching, the practitioner can first inform them of various ways to make disclosures. Role-play is useful for rehearsing various approaches to telling others and practicing a projected disclosure conversation (Gartrell, 1984; Mallon, 1998b). The practitioner and client can play both sides of an interchange, and the role-play can be audiotaped and played back for critique and revision (Kuehlwein, 1992).

Disclosures in Ethnic and Racial Families

The options for disclosure and the outcomes may vary depending on the context. For example, facilitating the disclosure process for persons from different ethnic and racial groups requires an understanding of their cultures (Rust, 1996a) and thoughts about what may happen following disclosure. This process is particularly difficult, for example, for Asian gay and lesbian persons. They may also be reluctant to seek out practitioners or support groups because of the stigma associated with seeking mental health services and the possible loss of confidentiality (Nakajima et al., 1996). In a study of Asian-American lesbian and gay persons who were seeing practitioners, Chan (1992) found that the most common themes identified by practitioners were the fear of rejection from families and the anticipation of a complete lack of understanding from parents. These clients need to be supported throughout the long process of gaining understanding and acceptance by their parents. Another task is to help them modify feelings of guilt for choosing a desired life that meets their own needs instead of what their parents want. The dilemma is how to be an adult with one's own needs and yet continue as a part of the family.

Latino lesbian and gay persons must prepare for the possibility that their families may never understand their lives and that many of them, particularly gay persons, will feel alienated within the Latino community. The practitioner in contact with the family can emphasize the Latino values of respecting all family members and the family's dedication to loyalty (Morales, 1996).

When working with gay and lesbian Native Americans, acculturation and the corresponding cultural values and conflict in allegiances need to be addressed. If these clients are having trouble coping with conflicts in allegiances, finding ways in which they can begin to integrate their disparate worlds may help. Native American organizations and support groups can assist with this goal. Additional sources of assistance are most likely necessary if clients are not acculturated. This involves drafting other members of their families or tribes as well as elders or medicine persons to help them achieve a positive identity. Other interventions include access to positive Native American role models specific to clients' Native American culture and tribe, and involvement with more gay and lesbian persons. It is crucial for Native American clients to find culturally relevant ways to come out and make disclosures that do not deny the gay or lesbian or the Native American aspects of themselves (K. L. Walters, 1997).

African-American LGB persons may not disclose to their families because their families tend to discourage disclosure of a non-heterosexual identity. Chapter 2 presented many reasons that underlie the negative responses to disclosures in African-American families and communities. Yet not all families are rejecting if, for example, LGB family members do not make an issue of their sexual orientation (M. A. Jones & Hill, 1996). African-American LGB persons face decisions similar to other ethnic and racial LGB persons. They should weigh the pros and cons of making disclosures and negotiate between their parents' desires and their own desires to not deny who they are.

Ethnic and racial persons must contend with the external systemic factors of heterosexism and racism and the internal issues of resolving conflicting allegiances. Practitioners should focus on the resilience and positive coping of these persons and reinforce a positive sense of an integrated self. These and other LGB persons need to be reminded of their strengths (K. L. Walters, 1997).

Disclosures at Work

Discrimination in the workplace makes the disclosure of a LGBT identity difficult. Cost-benefit analyses of disclosures can be useful in most contexts, including work settings. Compare the likely benefits of disclosure (for example, honesty, support, preventing any possibility of blackmail, bringing partners to work events) to the possible costs (for example, lost income, demotions, job loss, no promotions, deprecation, gossip, social isolation, harassment) (M. Pope, 1996; Vargo, 1998). A person with a larger income may think the costs of disclosure are high compared to the benefits of no disclosure. A person with a lower income may think that the costs of disclosure are lower when compared to the benefits (Badgett, 1996), unless they are the sole source of income or do not have a good chance of getting another job.

Before she began making disclosures on her job, Deevey (1993) wrote a plan using the assessment and planning skills she learned in nursing school. She identified plus factors for disclosure, such as nurses whose support she could seek and potential areas of difficulty such as a lack of positive role models and potential condemnation from closeted lesbian friends. Following disclosure in the workplace, Vargo (1998) cautioned that one must prepare for the possibility of being treated differently from other workers. If mistreatment is likely, one should learn in advance the protections and nondiscrimination policies of the workplace.

Transgender persons may have a particularly hard time holding jobs (Anderson, 1998). Disclosures at work are usually a last step for these persons, after taking hormones for a long time, living most of their time outside the workplace in the sex-gender they are adopting, and obtaining a legal name change. It is best to deal with many other issues before addressing issues resulting from disclosures at work. The results of hormonal intervention, however, can have rapid effects in some persons. A beard or breasts may develop so quickly that a more rapid outing at work might occur. A lower dosage of hormones may slow down these developments (Cole et al., 2000).

SUMMARY

In helping midlife and older persons during coming out, practitioners can use developmental models of coming out (e.g., SIF and the dual branch models) but with the realization that not everyone follows the steps in sequence. Information on community services and support groups will also be important. The same guidelines apply when working with bisexual clients, although they may experience even more confusion about what is happening than gay and lesbian persons. This is due to many myths about bisexuality, including such beliefs that it does not exist or is a temporary state. Other complications ensue because often it is only one partner who is bisexual and the other person must cope with having a nonmonogomous partner. Negotiated contracts are helpful. When LGB clients want assistance with disclosures, practitioners can help them decide who will be more inclined to accept the information well and suggest that disclosures happen with them first. They can also advise when disclosures are best made and where, and how to present the information. Practitioners must be sensitive to the cultural and religious beliefs of racial and ethnic families, and the difficulties these beliefs can create for a lesbian, gay, or bisexual family member ready to disclose. In the workplace, as in other settings, a cost-benefit analysis of disclosures is useful.

Chapter 10

Practice with Couples and Families

Competent practice with lesbian and gay couples and families begins with accurate knowledge. Same-sex couples and families are similar to heterosexual couples and families. Yet they experience unique obstacles because of heterosexism. Unfortunately, practitioners may also exhibit heterosexual bias in how they approach these couples and families (Gonsiorek & Weinrich, 1991; Markowitz, 1991).

The Committee on Lesbian and Gay Concerns of the American Psychological Association (APA) reported that there are many biased practitioners working with lesbian and gay couples. For example, they may ask members in a couple who plays the male role and who plays the female role, a question most lesbian and gay couples would respond to with disbelief. They do not value these couples or the members' commitment to each other. They may tell a couple to view their difficulties as insurmountable and encourage dissolution. They may also presume that their families are inappropriate. They may not provide or recommend any services (Garnets et al., 1991).

Work with lesbian and gay couples should follow the guidelines of exemplary practice identified by the Committee on Lesbian and Gay Concerns (APA, 1991): (1) have knowledge about the diverse nature of lesbian and gay relationships and validate their importance; (2) recognize the effects of prejudice and discrimination on lesbian and gay relationships and parenting; and (3) recognize the importance of alternative families for lesbian and gay persons (Garnets et al., 1991).

It is also important to view lesbian and gay couples on individual terms as they are quite varied. This can can include differences in duration of relationships, current developmental issues or concerns, living arrangements, economic situations, distribution of resources and power, degree of sexual and emotional exclusivity, adoption of traditional or more contemporary relationship models, and the presence or absence of children.

Practitioners may need to help once-married lesbians adapt to differences between heterosexual marriage with males and a relationship with another woman. Bridges and Croteau (1994) identified several of these differences: lack of social validation for lesbian couples, perhaps more difficulty negotiating the balance between autonomy and connection, and differences in sexual practices such as more emphasis on kissing and hugging versus goal-oriented orgasms.

Midlife and older couples may bring many other issues to practitioners including competition, power, overseparation, autonomy, too much closeness, sexuality, safe sex, and effects of HIV/AIDS on gay couples (see Hunter & Hickerson, 2003, for discussions of these issues). Several other issues, internalized oppression and identity development and disclosures, are discussed here. In addition, the importance of social support is discussed and legal protections for couples are identified.

ISSUES INVOLVING INTERNALIZED OPPRESSION

When a practitioner first sees a gay or lesbian couple, the couple will probably seem, on the surface, affirmative about their sexual orientation (APA, 1991). The oppression of heterosexism, however, can operate in subtle and nonconscious ways, and even persons with positive self-images are not totally shielded from this oppression (L. S. Brown, 1996). For example, some persons devalue same-sex intimacy, setting themselves up for failure in relationships. Some partners think that since they will eventually break up, they should never combine anything. For the same reason, some partners may establish loose boundaries for their links. Other couples may tighten their boundaries and become closed systems. Such systems, however, put much pressure on the couple partners to fulfill most of each other's needs (L. S. Brown, 1996; McVinney, 1998).

If internalized oppression is an issue for one or both partners, it should be the first focus for intervention. Practitioners need to challenge these couples' assumptions and expectations for failure (Okun, 1996). They need to communicate to these couples that the choice of a gay or lesbian partner is as natural as the choice of a heterosexual partner (Igartua, 1998). Practitioners can connect couples with support groups to meet other lesbian and gay couples who overcame issues associated with internalized oppression. If such groups are not available, affirmative and educational books and videos are useful (MacDonald, 1998). Groups are preferable, however, because although establishing boundaries between themselves and the outside world may be necessary, group contact will help these couples build social networks (Laird, 1996).

ISSUES INVOLVING IDENTITY DEVELOPMENT AND DISCLOSURE

Couple members may be at different stages in identity development and at different levels of comfort with disclosures. Questions to consider include: How "out" is each partner? How out is the couple? Who are they out to, or not out to, and in what contexts (Cabaj & Klinger, 1996)? Couples may fight over whether to disclose to parents or at work, or the exclusion of a partner from family and work social events (L. S. Brown, 1996).

The partner who has made more progress in identity development and disclosure may be patient and tolerant or impatient and frustrated about the other partner's "immaturity." Practitioners can provide each partner a clearer view of the other's unique experiences (L. S. Brown, 1996). For example, a partner who wants to be more open must understand the other partner's fear of possibly losing friends, job, and family (MacDonald, 1998). Practitioners must also challenge the notion that one partner's desire for openness or secrecy is symbolic of love, or not, for the other partner. Love and disclosure are independent of each other (Roth, 1985).

BENEFITS OF SOCIAL SUPPORT

Social support can be essential for lesbian and gay couples in relational adjustments and in the reduction of relational distress (Greene, 1994; Kurdek, 1988a,b; Kurdek & Schmitt, 1987). In a sample of 156 cohabiting gay couples, R. G. Smith and Brown (1998) found that social support for the couples was significantly associated with the quality of their linkups and strengthening the commitment of the partners. Persons in the social network may encourage the couple to stay together through stressful times. Practitioners should emphasize the benefits of social support and encourage couples to participate in interactions with friends, as well as family. Formal groups can also provide opportunities for lesbian and gay couples to meet and offer each other support, practical as well as emotional.

LEGAL PROTECTIONS IN THE EVENT OF SERIOUS ILLNESS, DEATH, OR BREAKUP

Lesbian and gay couples may need to protect themselves from others, possibly heterosexist family members or social institutions. For example, if one of the partners dies, the surviving partner may think that because of the other partners' desires, he or she will inherit various assets of that partner. Families of the deceased partner, however, often intervene and even overturn wills that left property to a partner (Vetri, 1998). There are no legal protections regarding inheritance laws, except those which lesbian and gay partners obtain themselves (e.g, trusts, durable powers of attorney, wills, and legal evidence of co-ownership) (Mail, 2002).

Practitioners need to discuss with couples the need for written documents, identified by Kuehlwein and Gottschalk (2000), that will allow the partners to

1. create joint financial arrangements;
2. inherit the house if the other partner dies;
3. be the chief beneficiaries of each other's will;
4. make medical decisions for the other in a medical crisis;
5. make decisions in a financial crisis;
6. develop instructions for medical intervention in the event of irreversible coma or terminal illness of a partner;
7. develop instructions for what should happen to a partner's body in case of death;
8. designate the partners as equal coparents of children;
9. designate the surviving partner as guardian to children; and
10. designate another guardian for the children if both partners die.

The idea is to ensure that a couple has made the legal and economic provisions they desire if needed.

Several specific examples of protections include

1. a *contract of love* that covers the joint payment of outstanding debts and distribution of personal and real property acquired during and before the link (Robson, 1995);
2. a *general power of attorney* that allows one to make and implement decisions about a partner's property and related matters if partner is no longer competent to do so (Baron & Cramer, 2000);
3. a *medical directive/living will* that allows a partner to determine desires about medical treatment and pain management in advance (Gruskin, 1999);
4. a *health care power of attorney* that prevents being barred from hospital access to one's partner, being prohibited from involvement in medical decisions for an incapacitated partner, and having no right to be the guardian for an incapacitated partner (Vetri, 1998);
5. a *conservatoryship/guardianship* that allows a person to specify wishes for the partner to make personal and business decisions in the event of incapacitation;
6. a *last will and testament* that allows a person to choose what happens to property and children in the event of death (without a will all property and sometimes joint property goes to relatives);
7. if available, a *stand-by guardian* appointed by a terminally ill partner who determines under what circumstances and by whom any children will be cared for upon death;
8. *funeral arrangements* that allow what the partner wanted; and
9. a *living trust* that provides a way to avoid probate (a court proceeding) (Gruskin, 1999; L. M. Woolf, 2002).

Although practitioners cannot give legal counsel, they need to know about these various legal protections. They should also have a list of legal resources available for clients, as well as books and Web sites (Kuehlwein & Gottschalk, 2000). To protect as much personal, medical, and property rights as possible, planning should begin in midlife (Humphreys & Quam, 1998).

There should also be agreements made in advance in case of a breakup. Separation distress is the same for all couples going through a breakup (Kurdek, 1997). Interventions for grieving heterosexual partners, then, are applicable to lesbian and gay couples. The differences are that when lesbian and gay partnerships dissolve, no legal guidelines govern the division of property. Resolution of disputes depends upon on the goodwill of the partners. Because partners in dissolved relationships do not always have goodwill (Hartman, 1996), same sex-gender couples should prepare an accord in advance of separation. This agreement can include how the couple will divide property that they bought together and other merged assets. With a formal financial strategy to specify how to divide property and other resources, couples are less likely to experience an acrimonious dispute (Chambers, 1998). If none of these agreements exist, mediation is an alternative (Hartman, 1996).

ISSUES EXPERIENCED BY COUPLES
WITH BISEXUAL MEMBERS

When one or both members of a couple identifies as bisexual, practice becomes even more complex. Similar to work with couples on any issue, the practitioner should evaluate the general strength and flexibility of the relationship, patterns of interaction and roles, partners' satisfaction with the relationship and the quality of the couple's sexual life, communication skills, conflict-resolution skills and deficits, and the presence of other or unresolved couple issues or stressors. Additional considerations for bisexual couples, suggested by Paul (1992), include the heterosexism or biphobia of each partner and the supports available to both partners.

Based on the work of Deacon, Reinke, and Viers (1998), the issues that bisexual clients and their heterosexual partners might want to work on can be divided into behavioral, cognitive, and affective categories. In the *behavioral* category, potential issues include alteration of the family structure; disclosure to children, family, and friends; integration of a gay or lesbian partner into the marriage; feelings of rejection and betrayal by one's marital partner; and the use of money for outside relationships (Buxton, 1994). Couples may need to learn problem-solving skills to work out a new structure and set of rules (Deacon et al., 1998). Once a bisexual partner begins experiencing sex outside the primary link, sexual difficulties may arise within the primary link that may also need to be addressed (Coleman, 1985a). In the *cognitive* category, issues can include perceptions of sexual identity, assumptions regarding discrimination and internalized oppression, standards regarding monogamy and multiple partners, and attributions and automatic thoughts such as blaming relationship difficulties on a partner's bisexual orientation. In the *affective* category, issues include depression and anger over unfulfilled desires and jealousy over outside relationships (Deacon et al., 1998). Several of these issues and examples of interventions are discussed in the following.

A key issue in working with mixed-orientation couples is the jealousy of the monogamous partner. Jealousy is rooted in a sense of insecurity or fear of losing the relationship (Matteson, 1996a). Bisexual attractions in one of the partners raise understandable issues of insecurity in the other partner, even when the underlying relationship is strong. The bisexual person's partner recognizes that she or he cannot compete with a potential partner of the other sex-gender (Stokes & Damon, 1995). A constructive focus would be to explore what the bisexual partner can do to clarify his or her commitment to the primary link (Matteson, 1996a). Rarely can a couple with a bisexual member shift the marriage from a traditional one to an open relationship without agreements that the marital partner will remain primary to the bisexual partner (M. S. Weinberg et al., 1994). The couple should discuss the primacy of the marriage and their commitment to it (Coleman, 1985b). Still, open relationships are difficult to maintain and often falter because of inability to handle the complexity of demands, jealousy issues, and the lack of social support (Matteson, 1995).

Commitment of the couple members and satisfaction with their relationship can empower them to act on pertinent issues. These couples may need help in slowing down and reducing the pressure for an instantaneous resolution of all the complications; a moratorium period permits necessary communication, reflection, education, and moving beyond the initial emotional upset (Paul, 1992).

When ready, couples with a nomonogamous partner need to work out a new structure and accompanying rules. Many can develop stable, satisfying relationships via contracts. A couple can develop a detailed and individually tailored contract with ground rules and explicit guidelines for what the partners can and cannot do with relationships outside the marriage. Practitioners can assist with contract writing and negotiate what to include. The contract must elucidate safe-sex practices and there should be no unilateral secrets. All rules should be readily open to discussion and revision. Some heterosexual partners want to know about the bisexual partner's sexual activities with others and this is agreed upon between the partners (Matteson, 1995; Paul, 1992). Other couples may have no explicit discussion of these activities, maintaining secrets about outside sexual activities. The practitioner should challenge the couples to have no secrets (Matteson, 1995).

Practitioners may assist a bisexual marriage partner in balancing multiple partners. No matter what the arrangements between the partners, however, this is not an easy task. It requires communication skills, trust between partners, and the ability of the heterosexual partner to handle jealousy. It also requires skill in time management (Paul, 1992). Often, when a bisexual person seeks a practitioner, the relationship balance is destabilized by internal or external stressors (Matteson, 1996a).

HIV/AIDS

The issue of HIV/AIDS applies to both bisexual and gay persons, especially if they are not committed to monogamy (Stokes et al., 1998). Some HIV-positive men do not always disclose their status to sexual partners, including steady ones. Some think that disclosure is unnecessary because they use condoms. Practitioners should take a strong exception to this practice because all partners, whether bisexual, heterosexual, gay, or lesbian, have the right to decide if the risk is acceptable for them. If regular intercourse occurs without a condom or without disclosure, the practitioner should insist that the client inform partners. If the client refuses, "duty-to-protect" laws in some states require practitioners to notify persons who unknowingly are at physical risk by the client's behavior (Matteson, 1996a). Yet these laws may be ambiguous about their applicability to the practice of safe sex. Before informing partners, therefore, practitioners should consult other practitioners and obtain legal counsel (Hughes & Friedman, 1994; Marks, 1993).

FAMILIES

Generally, practitioners intervene with lesbian and gay families as they do with all families. Yet, although lesbian and gay parents have as many social skills and psychological strengths as heterosexual parents, they live in an environment hostile to them and they do not have suitable legal protection for themselves or their families (Gonsiorek, 1996). Heterosexual parents receive assistance from formalized support systems, but lesbian and gay parents do not get this support (e.g., C. J. Patterson, 1994, 1995; Ricketts & Achtenberg, 1990).

Lesbian and gay parents also get mixed support from their families of origin. Even when the family of origin is somewhat accepting or tolerant of one's sexual orientation and even of the couple's relationship, reactions may change if the couple decides to raise children. Members of one's family of origin may act on the myths they learned about psychological and social difficulties the children are thought to experience (Ariel & Sterns, 1992; Matthews & Lease, 2000). Some family members think it is wrong for a gay or lesbian couple to bring a child into what they see as a sinful relationship (Muzio, 1999). Yet for some lesbian and gay couples having children brings them closer to their extended families, as having children may afford them more mainstream status. Family members sometimes rally to support the couple and are available for and attentive to the children (Gartrell et al., 1999). Two-thirds of a sample of thirty-one lesbians with children studied by Nations (1997) rated family support as moderately high to high.

Few communities openly endorse lesbian and gay families, although some extend less hostility and fewer obstacles so these families are not harassed. Urban settings are more tolerant than rural ones (Friedman, 1997). Lesbian and gay families usually have less support from their own communities than heterosexual families receive. Lesbian and gay communities are not as structured around children as are heterosexual communities. When heterosexual mothers experience the arrival of a child, they feel integrated into their communities whereas lesbian mothers feel more isolated or more like a "separate" family (Stiglitz, 1990). Because of the increased rate of lesbian and gay couples who are parents, however, support systems among these couples are expanding (Scrivner & Eldridge, 1995).

Children

In general, families headed by lesbian mothers or gay fathers seem remarkably similar to heterosexual families in their concerns and parent-child relationships. Practitioners need to be informed, however, that these families are charting new territory, which undoubtedly creates stress for them. A. Martin's (1993) *The Lesbian and Gay Parenting Handbook* is an excellent resource, offering extensive lists of resources across the nation as well as practical advice about adoption, disclosure, and family life. This detailed guide can help both practitioner and clients. Other useful resources include *For Lesbian Parents* (S. M. Johnson & O'Connor, 2001), *The Queer Parent's Primer* (Brill, 2001), and *The Lesbian Parenting Book: A Guide to Creating Families and Raising Children* (Clunis & Green, 2003). It is helpful to provide children with a general explanation about two persons of the same sex-gender caring for each other. Various books are useful to educate them, for example, *Daddy's Roommate* (Willhoite, 2000).

Because society does not generally recognize lesbian and gay families, it is especially important for these families to develop rituals, traditions, and other ways to celebrate family successes (Laird, 1994). It is also important to connect with other lesbian and gay families so they can feel that their family is not unusual. The practitioner should emphasize the need for both celebrations and interchanges with other lesbian and gay families. Parents, Families and Friends of Lesbians and Gays (PFLAG) is a resource available in many communities to support families and children. PFLAG is available online at <http://www.pflag.org>. Another Web site for LGBT couples and families that provides information about services and resources is <http/www.altfamily.org>.

SUMMARY

Gay and lesbian partners must negotiate similar tasks faced by heterosexual couples by living together and, sometimes, raising a family together. Often, practitioners can employ the same techniques. Yet, certain practice issues are unique to gay and lesbian couples, such as coming out and disclosures. In addition, internalized oppression resulting from heterosexism can affect couples in several ways: devaluing of same sex-gender relationships, thinking that same sex-gender relationships cannot last, and tightening the boundaries around a couple so that the partners are the only ones meeting each other's needs. Support from other couples is helpful. Because of the lack of legal protections that are automatic for heterosexual couples, lesbian and gay couples must seek out their own legal protections in case serious illness, death of a partner, or a breakup occurs. As suggested earlier, bisexual couples are complex and will have many issues to deal with as well as work out rules and contracts. Practice with gay and lesbian families with children will often focus on support resources and advocacy. One of the major roles practitioners can take with these families is that of an advocate in heterosexist institutions.

Chapter 11

Group and Community Practice with Older Lesbian and Gay Persons

As LGBT persons grow older, they rely more on public programs and social services for care and assistance. This most likely means less independence from heterosexist institutions (Cahill et al., 2000) in which they may not even be welcome. For example, openly lesbian and gay persons are not welcome in senior centers in New York City (National Gay and Lesbian Task Force Policy Institute, 2000). Of particular concern is what happens to a transgender person with a noncongruent body (an uninformed observer may think that the genitals or other physical features of a person do not match the gender and/or legal identity). What will happen when this person has to be intimately assisted by health care providers and caregivers, such as with bathing?

TWO MODELS FOR SERVICES

It is important to develop affirmative programs to meet the desires of older lesbian and gay persons. Two models for services for older lesbian and gay persons were identified by Tully (2000). First, the separate but equal model such as SAGE in New York City believes to ensure appropriate services are provided, they must be developed and implemented by the lesbian and gay community. This model has been the prevalent one since the 1970s and remains an important way to provide social services for older lesbian and gay persons. This population prefers to use social and support services provided in lesbian and gay programs, but such organizations do not always exist. Disadvantages to this model include the necessity of being open about sexual orientation to obtain these services.

The second model requires appropriate services for older lesbian and gay persons be provided in the more traditional social services agencies in which openness is not an issue. Social work administrators can develop programs in mainstream agencies once they learn what is needed for specialized, functional, and accessible social services for this population. Through a diverse array of media, SAGE invests considerable effort educating professional communities and the general public about the needs of older lesbian and gay persons in a wide variety of settings. SAGE advocates for more sensitive services delivery, support, and advocacy. In-service training programs at local agencies sensitize staff to the issues and needs of these persons. Information is disseminated at conferences, and a speaker's bureau provides leaders for panels and group discussions. Educational materials are published in newsletters and magazines and broadcast on television and radio (R. J. Jacobs, Rasmussen, & Hohman, et al., 1999). The disadvantages of this model are that most traditional agencies are not consulted by SAGE or other lesbian and gay organizations. Their employees will likely assume that all clients are heterosexual and treat them as such and will be ill equipped to provide services to older lesbian and gay persons.

Because of the heterosexism in traditional services, developing more affirmative services for older lesbian and gay persons is crucial. Programs that work to eliminate bias among service providers to these older persons are vital to the development of a safe, comfortable aging process (Cahill et al., 2000). Services such as outreach programs must acknowledge and respect fears of older persons who never came out of the closet. It is always their choice whether to participate (Reid, 1995).

In working with older lesbian and gay persons, it is particularly important for human services professionals to move beyond the training they might have received in individual, intrapsychic approaches to the use of advocacy and consultative interventions. For example, they can be human services brokers and connect older lesbian and gay clients with agencies and service providers that support gay rights and are sensitive to the special needs and concerns of these persons. They also should be knowledgeable about the resources available in the LGBT communities (Faria, 1997). Service delivery and program design should always begin with a clear understanding of the expectations of those whom the services will serve. Many older lesbian and gay persons will also be resources (e.g., money and talents) for some of the needed services (Shenk & Fullmer, 1996).

The community organizing and group services approach offers more promise of meeting the needs of this population than the direct provision of specific services. When asked what their greatest human need was, most of the gay persons studied by L. B. Brown et al. (1997) indicated acceptance, validation, and love from others. In an assessment of needs among older lesbian and gay persons in Chicago, Beeler et al. (1999) discovered that expanded opportunities to socialize with other older lesbian and gay persons were by far the most commonly expressed need. In addition, the respondents wanted social opportunities other than bars.

Expanded social opportunities might be an especially acute desire for gay persons who have lost many close friends and partners to AIDS, and for men and women who came out later in life and want to develop a network of lesbian and gay friends. Others who felt they would benefit from expanded social opportunities also wanted a focus on social activities and social interactions that are not age stratified. Some who did not yet think of themselves as the older generation wanted to meet retired persons so they could picture what retired life might eventually be like for them. They were hoping for reassurance that retirement was a positive experience (Beeler et al., 1999).

Various group services can meet the needs for support and social/recreational involvements as well as provide counseling, education, and advocacy. Specific benefits of groups, identified by Fassinger (1997), include

1. *affiliation,* for example, countering isolation;
2. *affirmation,* for example, understanding one's feelings about a lost partner;
3. *universality,* for example, normalizing one's experiences;
4. *ventilation/catharsis,* for example, talking about and expressing feelings about issues in one's life;
5. *integration,* for example, integrating sexual orientation into one's overall identity;
6. *altruism and meaningful roles,* for example, mentoring, sharing knowledge and skills;
7. *socializing techniques and interpersonal learning,* for example, using others as guides for transitions, benefitting from hearing about their experiences; and

8. *information, resources, and problem solving,* for example, learning about community resources and how to access them.

Frost (1997) also recommended a group setting for gay persons to help combat isolation resulting from losses, to examine myths and stereotypes about aging, and to develop deeper nonsexual relationships with other gay persons. Gay persons prefer groups unmixed in sexual orientation.

Human services professionals may need to replace or expand on their role as a direct provider of group services. More effective roles would be as a consultant or supervisor in setting up self-help groups in a community. Advocacy for other social services is also important for older lesbian and gay clients (Fassinger, 1997), once this population has identified the services they need.

The Chicago sample of older lesbian and gay persons (Beeler et al., 1999) expressed other needs in addition to social opportunities:

- *Giving back:* There was a desire to give back to the lesbian and gay community and to become more involved in the community. This was also a way to meet others.
- *Volunteer registry:* A volunteer registry would provide names, phone numbers, and other information of lesbian and gay adults in the community.
- *Support groups:* Support groups would be for persons in similar situations such as gay fathers or for those who were heterosexually married, divorced, and then came out. "Support" also overlapped with the desire for additional social opportunities. In a San Diego sample studied by R. J. Jacobs and colleagues (1999), both men and women used lesbian and gay social and support groups more often than other types of services provided by the lesbian and gay community.
- *Counseling services:* Counseling services were desired only when they focused on particular situations, such as disclosure to children or developmental transitions such as retirement or the death of a partner. The respondents did not want "treatment." Mental health needs were the least indicated needs.
- *Information and education:* More information and education were desired.

- *Workshops and seminars:* Workshops and seminars were wanted on various topics of interest such as estate planning, retirement finances, and legal issues focusing on topics such as wills and powers of attorney.
- *Advocacy:* Advocacy services would include training and educating mainstream services providers to be sensitive to the needs of lesbian and gay clients.
- *Referral network:* This would be a link to services, programs, and events through an information and referral system created specifically for older lesbian and gay persons. The focus of the referral network would be lesbian and gay-friendly providers for older-adult services, such as health care facilities, attorneys, nursing homes, and in-home health care providers.
- *Basic needs:* Some older lesbian and gay persons needed food, shelter, and medical care. Some also needed transportation to participate in any program. Some might need help with basic household tasks to continue living independently. These various needs suggested the development of a case management program to assist these particular older lesbian and gay persons in procuring suitable services.
- *Outreach program:* An outreach program was needed to target isolated persons and those unable to locate services agencies.

COMMUNITY ORGANIZING ON BEHALF OF OLDER LESBIAN AND GAY PERSONS

Separate services for aging lesbian and gay persons were recommended by Quam and Whitford (1992). Association with others with the same sexual orientation and similar concerns increases the likelihood of acceptance of aging and high life satisfaction. Social services organizations based on the separate-but-equal model for older lesbian and gay persons are growing in the United States and Canada to meet these needs. Several organizations in large urban areas provide comprehensive social and support services. The most comprehensive program is Senior Action in a Gay Environment (SAGE) in New York (Friend, 1987; Grenwald, 1984). For more programs see Chapter 3.

The population of older lesbian and gay persons is diverse, presents a large range of needs as in the previous list, and often benefits from a variety of services. Unfortunately, comprehensive organizations that could meet such a large range of needs are not feasible in most locations. The array of services offered by SAGE is beyond the capacity of any single agency or even several agencies that usually compete for limited resources. A community-based approach may be a solution to this situation, as it would draw upon the substantial and varied resources of the target population itself. Time, energy, and funds would be directed toward organizing older lesbian and gay persons. They can help one another and provide needed services for each other (Beeler et al., 1999).

A community organizing approach involves older lesbian and gay persons in the identification, planning, and implementation of a variety of services. For example, as noted, older lesbian and gay persons identified the needs for more opportunities to socialize with other lesbian and gay persons and to become involved in meaningful community activities. Meeting these needs might be best realized through an organization or community center in which older lesbian and gay persons not only are the recipients of services but are also actively engaged in the provision of services. Many members of this population possess an array of talents and resources, including knowledge, expertise, skills, experience, time, and money. Respondents (Beeler et al., 1999) expressed a willingness to dedicate themselves and some combination of resources to helping others. This approach also helps alleviate the most frequently cited need encountered: additional opportunities for meaningful community involvement and social interactions with other lesbian and gay persons.

Three key components necessary in the "community organization approach" were identified by Beeler et al. (1999) as (1) resources for developing a forum in which older lesbian and gay persons can become involved in identifying, planning, organizing, and providing services; (2) a volunteer registry of services and programs developed, organized, and maintained by volunteers; and (3) some means for coordinating various agencies and organizations within the community to prevent duplication of services. Goals identified by Beeler et al. for serving older lesbian and gay persons, based on the aforementioned needs assessment presented, are as follows:

- *To provide ongoing opportunities for social interaction and opportunities to build friendship networks and create or expand existing supports:* Expand involvement in the LGB community by social, educational, and fun activities structured so that persons can talk to each other before leaving the events. Social events can include dances, brunches, picnics, potluck lunches, day trips, workshops, and rap groups; also provide opportunities for some sex-gender specific or sex-gender segregated activities.
- *To provide information and discussion opportunities:* Include support groups and activity groups that encourage sharing of feelings, concerns, interests, and special issues. Educational workshops can be hosted on a variety of topics such as dating, starting a relationship, how to maintain and end relationships, and abusive relationships. Examples of the focus for other groups include coming out, bereavement, and peer counseling. Groups can also focus on personal growth, creative writing, language, history projects, and books.
- *To create an information and referral system of services and programs and events:* Tailor this specifically for older lesbian and gay persons and include information lines for resources, services, programs and events, referrals to legal services, and lesbian and gay physicians.
- *To provide a resource manual:* List services, doctor and other practitioner referrals, legal assistance, programs, publications, churches and temples, and other resources, updated on a monthly basis. Such a manual would be useful for all older lesbian and gay persons and for counselors, phone hotline volunteers, and crisis counselors. A monthly newsletter with a calendar of events and a schedule of support and activity groups can be sent to consumers and other agencies. Volunteers can fold newsletters and stuff envelopes at monthly "mailing parties."
- *To provide outreach services:* Maintain services for persons who are homebound or living in nursing homes, persons living in rural areas, and persons who feel isolated. Examples of outreach services include a "buddy system" visiting program for persons living on their own who are frail, ill, or otherwise housebound or socially isolated. These persons can receive LGB-oriented newspapers and opportunities to correspond with other

LGB persons. Direct contact can be supplemented with telephone contact.

- *To establish a networking system:* Ensure accountability of services providers and quality of care and services by including other agencies.
- *To provide assistance in procuring fair and adequate services:* This includes health care, legal assistance, and financial assistance.

Other resources for older lesbian and gay persons are Internet addresses: Lesbian and Gay Issues Network (www.asaging.org), a constituent group of the American Society on Aging; and Senior Pride Network (www.pridesenior.org). Both have extensive Web sites with resources and links for older lesbian and gay persons. The Gay and Lesbian Association of Retiring Persons (GLARP) (www. gaylesbian retiring.org) provides an alternative to other related organizations that may not recognize or work for the needs of older lesbian and gay persons (L. M. Woolf, 2002). PrideNet has a resource list for older LGBT persons with links to several areas of interest (http://www. pridenet.com/senior.htm). The Senior Cyborgs also have a useful homepage that has chat rooms, library resources, information about disabilities, legal links, home and garden tips, insurance information, meeting spots, pets, and topics related to death and dying (http:// www.online96.com/seniors/gay.html).

USE OF SOCIAL SERVICES

Older lesbian and gay participants studied by R. J. Jacobs et al. (1999) in San Diego used social and support groups within the lesbian and gay community, but also used general community health services. They rated lesbian and gay services in their city as more adequate in meeting needs in times of emotional crises than nonlesbian and nongay services. Future utilization of social services among the respondents was also addressed. About one-third (32 percent) said they would participate once a week in programs for older lesbian and gay persons; 20 percent every other week; and 25 percent once a month. Some (9 percent) would participate more than once a week. Nearly half (49 percent) would never participate in lesbian and gay programs within nonlesbian and gay organizations. Both women and men indicated that they would be interested in participating in social groups within the lesbian and gay community segregated by sex-gender. About one-third (31 percent) would never participate in mixed sex-gender social programs; 41 percent would participate but only once a month. When asked what types of programs or social services they would like to see available, the respondents requested social and support groups more than any other services. About one-third said they would use phone contact services, bereavement groups, and transportation services. Women (53 percent) were significantly more interested in bereavement groups than men (24 percent). Other types of services that older lesbian and gay persons would use if available included peer counseling, employment, dating, and help finding affordable housing.

SUMMARY

Older lesbian and gay persons must rely more on public programs and social services for care and assistance, with less independence from heterosexist institutions. It is important to develop affirmative programs to meet the needs of these older lesbian and gay persons. Such programs are based on two models for services: the separate but equal model like SAGE in New York City and the provision of services in more traditional social services agencies. The separate but equal model is preferred, but not many programs are based on this model because of the comprehensive requirements. Because of this, group services and community organizing on behalf of older lesbian and gay persons can be the best way to administer needed services and to use the talents among this population to provide some of these services.

References

Adam, B. D. (1987). *The rise of the gay and lesbian movement.* Boston: Twayne.

Adam, B. D. (1995). *The rise of a gay and lesbian movement.* Revised edition. New York: Twayne Publishers.

Adams, C. L., & Kimmel, D. C. (1997). Exploring the lives of older African American gay men. In B. Greene (Ed.), *Ethnic and cultural diversity among lesbians and gay men* (pp. 132-151). Thousand Oaks, CA: Sage Publications.

Adelman, M. (1977). A comparison of professionally employed lesbians and heterosexual women on the MMPI. *Archives of Sexual Behavior, 6,* 193-201.

Adelman, M. (1980). Adjustment of aging and styles of being gay: A study of elderly gay men and lesbians (Doctoral dissertation, The Wright Institute, Berkeley 1980). *Dissertation Abstracts International, 40.*

Adelman, M. (1986). *Long time passing.* Boston: Alyson Press.

Adelman, M. (1988). Quieting our fears: Lesbians and aging. *Outlook: National Lesbian and Gay Quarterly, 1,* 78-81.

Adelman, M. (1990). Stigma, gay lifestyles and adjustment to aging: A study of later-life gay men and lesbians. *Journal of Homosexuality, 20,* 7-32.

Adelman, M. (1991). Stigma, gay lifestyles, and adjustment to aging: A study of later-life gay men and lesbians. In J. A. Lee (Ed.), *Gay midlife and maturity* (pp. 1-32). Binghamton, NY: The Haworth Press.

Adelman, M. (Ed.) (2000). *Midlife lesbian relationships: Friends, lovers, children, and parents.* Binghamton, New York: Harrington Park Press.

Adleman, J., Berger, R., Boyd, M., Doublex, V., Freedman, M., Hubbard, W., Kight, M., Kochman, A., Meyer, M. K. Robinson, & Raphael, S. M. (1993). *Lambda gray.* North Hollywood, CA: Newcastle Publishing.

Ainslie, J., & Feltey, K. M. (1991). Definitions and dynamics of motherhood and family in lesbian communities. *Marriage & Family Review, 17,* 63-85.

Alexander, C. J. (1998). Treatment planning for gay and lesbian clients. *Journal of Gay & Lesbian Social Services, 8,* 95-106.

Almvig, C. (1982). *The invisible minority: Aging and lesbianism.* New York: Utica College of Syracuse University.

Altman, C. (1999). Gay and lesbian seniors: Unique challenges of coming out in later life. *Siecus Report, 27,* 14-17.

Alzheimer's Association. (1995). *Advocate guide to 1995 national policy priorities.* Washington, DC: Author.

American Psychological Association. (2001). *Publication manual of the American Psychological Association* (Fifth ed.). Washington, DC: Author.

American Psychological Association, Committee on Lesbian and Gay Concerns. (1991). Avoiding heterosexist bias in language. *American Psychologist, 46,* 937-974.

American Society on Aging, Lesbian and Gay Aging Issues Network. (2004). Housing. Available online at <http://www.asaging.org/networks/lgain/lgainlinks. cfm? category=hsg>.

Anderson, B. F. (1998). Therapeutic issues in working with transgendered clients. In D. Denny (Ed.), *Current concepts of transgendered identity* (pp. 215-226). New York: Garland.

APHA policy statement 9933 (2000). The need for acknowledging transgendered individuals within research and clinical practice. *American Journal of Public Health, 90,* 483-484.

Appleby, G. A., & Anastas, J. W. (1998). *Not just a passing phase: Social work with gay, lesbian, and bisexual people.* New York: Columbia University Press.

Ariel, J., & Stearns, S. M. (1992). Challenges facing gay and lesbian families. In S. H. Dworkin & F. J. Gutieírrez (Eds.), *Counseling gay men and lesbians: Journey to the end of the rainbow* (pp. 95-112). Alexandria, VA: American Association for Counseling and Development.

Badgett, M. V. L. (1996). Employment and sexual orientation: Disclosure and discrimination in the workplace. *Journal of Gay & Lesbian Social Services, 4,* 29-52.

Bailey, J. M. (1996). Gender identity. In R. C. Savin-Williams & K. M. Cohen (Eds.), *The lives of lesbians, gays, and bisexuals: Children to adults* (pp. 71-93). Ft. Worth, TX: Harcourt Brace.

Ball, S. (1994). A group model for gay and lesbian clients with chronic mental illness. *Social Work, 39,* 109-115.

Baron, A., & Cramer, D. W. (2000). Potential counseling concerns of aging lesbian, gay and bisexual clients. In R. M. Perez, K. A. DeBord, & K. J. Bieschke (Eds.), *Handbook of counseling and psychotherapy with lesbian, gay, and bisexual clients* (pp. 207-223). Washington, DC: American Psychological Association.

Barr, R. F., & Catts, S. V. (1974). Psychiatry opinion and homosexuality: A short report. *Journal of Homosexuality, 1,* 213-215.

Barrett, B. (1998). Gay and lesbian activism: A frontier in social advocacy. In C. C. Lee (Ed.), *Social action: A mandate for counselors* (pp. 84-98). Alexandria, VA: American Counseling Association.

Barron, J. (1996). Some issues in psychotherapy with gay and lesbian clients. *Psychotherapy, 33,* 611-616.

Baruch, G., & Brooks-Gunn, J. (1984). The study of women in midlife. In G. Baruch & J. Brooks-Gunn (Eds.), *Women in midlife* (pp. 1-8). New York: Plenum Press.

Baum, M. I. (1996). Gays and lesbians choosing to be parents. In C. J. Alexander (Ed.), *Gay and lesbian mental health: A sourcebook for practitioners* (pp. 113-126). Binghamton, NY: The Haworth Press.

Bayer, R. (1987). *Homosexuality and American psychiatry: The politics of diagnosis in lesbians, gay man, and the law* (Second ed.). Princeton, NJ: Princeton University Press.

Becker, C. S. (1988). *Broken ties: Lesbian ex-lovers.* Boston: Alyson Press.

Beeler, J. A., Rawls, T. W., Herdt, G. H., & Cohler, B. J. (1999). Needs of older lesbians and gay men in Chicago. *Journal of Gay & Lesbian Social Services, 9,* 31.

Bell, A. P., & Weinberg, M. S. (1978). *Homosexualities: A study of diversity among men and women.* New York: Simon & Schuster.

Bennett, K. C., & Thompson, N. L. (1990). Accelerated aging and male homosexuality: Australian evidence in a continuing debate. *Journal of Homosexuality, 20,* 65-75.

Berger, R. M. (1980). Psychological adaptation of the older homosexual male. *Journal of Homosexuality, 5,* 161-175.

Berger, R. M. (1982). The unseen minority: Older gays and lesbians. *Social Work, 27,* 236-242.

Berger, R. M. (1984). Realities of gay and lesbian aging. *Social Work, 29,* 57-62.

Berger, R. M. (1985) Rewriting a bad script: Older lesbians and gays. In H. Hidalgo, T. L. Peterson, & N. J. Woodman (Eds.). *Lesbian and gay issues: A resource manual for social workers* (pp. 53-59). Silver Spring, MD: NASW.

Berger, R. M. (1990). Men together: Understanding the gay couple. *Journal of Homosexuality, 19,* 31-49.

Berger, R. M. (1992). Research on older gay men: What we know, what we need to know. In N. J. Woodman, (Ed.), *Lesbian and gay lifestyles: A guide for counseling and education* (pp. 217-233). New York: Irvington.

Berger, R. M. (1996). *Gay and gray: The older homosexual man* (Second ed.). Binghamton, NY: The Haworth Press.

Berger, R. M., & Kelly, J. J. (1986a). Gay men. In H. Gochros, J. Gochros, & J. Fischer (Eds.), *Helping the sexually oppressed* (pp. 162-180). Englewood Cliffs, NJ: Prentice-Hall.

Berger, R. M., & Kelly, J. J. (1986b). Working with homosexuals of the older population. *Social Casework, 67,* 203-210.

Berger, R. M., & Kelly, J. J. (1996). Gay men: Overview. In R. J. Edwards (Ed.), *Encyclopedia of social work,* (Nineteenth ed.), (pp. 1064-1075). Washington, DC: NASW Press.

Berger, R. M., & Kelly, J. J. (2001). What are older gay men like? An impossible question? *Journal of Gay & Lesbian Social Services, 13,* 55-64.

Berkman, C., & Zinberg, J. G. (1997). Homophobia and heterosexism in social workers. *Social Work, 42,* 319-331.

Bernhard, L. A., & Applegate, J. M. (1999). Comparison of stress and stress management strategies between lesbian and heterosexual women. *Health Care for Women International, 20,* 355-347.

Bernstein, G. S. (1992). How to avoid heterosexual bias in language. *Behavior Therapist, 15,* 161.

Berrill, K. T. (1990). Anti-gay violence and victimization in the United States. *Journal of Interpersonal Violence, 5,* 274-294.

Berrill, K. T. (1992). Organizing against hate on campus: Strategies for activists. In G. M. Herek & K. T. Berrill (Eds.), *Hate crimes: Confronting violence against lesbians and gay men* (pp. 259-269). Newbury Park, CA: Sage Publications.

Bérubé, A. (1990). *Coming out under fire: The history of gay men and women in World War Two*. New York: Free Press.

Bigner, J. (1996). Working with gay fathers. In J. Laird & R. Green (Eds.), *Lesbians and gays in couples and families* (pp. 370-403). San Francisco: Jossey-Bass.

Birk, L. (1980). The myth of classic homosexuality: Views of a behavioral psychotherapist. In J. Marmor (Ed.), *Homosexual behavior: A modern reappraisal* (pp. 376-390). New York: Basic Books.

Blackwood, E. (1984). Sexuality and gender in certain Native American tribes: The case of the cross-gender females. *Signs, 10*, 27-42.

Blando, J. A. (2001). Twice hidden: Older gay and lesbian couples, friends, intimacy. *Generations, 25*, 87-90.

Blumstein, P., & Schwartz, P. (1983). *American couples*. New York: William Morrow.

Bockting, W. O. (1999). From construction to context: Gender through the eyes of the transgendered. *Siecus Report, 28*, 3-7.

Bohan, J. S. (1996). *Psychology and sexual orientation: Coming to terms*. New York: Routledge.

Bohan, J. S. & Russell, G. M. (1999). Conceptual frameworks. In J. S. Bohan & G. M. Russell (Eds.), *Conversations about psychology and sexual orientation* (pp. 11-30). New York: New York University Press.

Bonilla, J., & Porter, J. (1990). A comparison of Latino, black, and non-Hispanic white attitudes toward homosexuality. *Hispanic Journal of Behavioral Sciences, 12*, 437-452.

Borden, W. (1989). Life review as a therapeutic frame in the treatment of young adults with AIDS. *Health & Social Work, 14*, 253-259.

Borden, W. (1992). Narrative perspectives in psychosocial intervention following adverse life events. *Social Work, 37*, 135-141.

Boxer, A. M. (1997). Gay, lesbian, and bisexual aging into the twenty-first century: An overview and introduction. *Journal of Gay, Lesbian, and Bisexual Identity, 2*, 187-197.

Bozett, F. W. (1993). Gay fathers: A review of the literature. In L. D. Garnets & D. C. Kimmel (Eds.), *Psychological perspectives on lesbian and gay male experiences* (pp. 437-457). New York: Columbia University Press.

Bradford, J., & Ryan, C. (1987). *National lesbian health care survey: Mental health implications*. Washington, DC: National Lesbian and Gay Health Foundation.

Bradford, J., & Ryan, C. (1991). Who we are: Health concerns of middle-aged lesbians. In B. J. Warshow, & A. J. Smith (Eds.), *Lesbians at midlife: The creative transition* (pp.147-163). San Francisco: Spinsters Book Company.

Bridges, K. L., & Croteau, J. M. (1994). Once-married lesbians: Facilitating changing life patterns. *Journal of Counseling and Development, 73*, 134-140.

Brill, S. A. (2001). *The queer parent's primer: A lesbian and gay families' guide to navigating the straight world*. Oakland, CA: New Harbinger.

Brown, G. R. (1998). Women in the closet: Relationships with transgendered men. In D. Denny (Ed.), *Current concepts of transgendered identity* (pp. 353-371). New York: Garland.

Brown, L. B. (1997). Women and men, not-men and not-women, lesbians and gays: American Indian gender-style alternatives. *Journal of Gay and Lesbian Social Services, 6,* 5-20.

Brown, L. B., Alley, G. R., Sarosy, S., Quarto, G., & Cook, T. (2001). Gay men: Aging well! *Journal of Gay & Lesbian Social Services, 13,* 41-54.

Brown, L. B., Sarosy, S. G., Cook, T. C., & Quarto, J. G. (1997). *Gay men and aging.* New York: Garland.

Brown, L. S. (1989). Lesbians, gay men and their families: Common clinical issues. *Journal of Gay & Lesbian Psychotherapy, 1,* 65-77.

Brown, L. S. (1995). Therapy with same-sex couples: An introduction. In N. S. Jacobson & A. S. Guttman (Eds.), *Clinical handbook of couple therapy* (pp. 274-291). New York: Guilford Press.

Brown, L. S. (1996). Ethical concerns with sexual minority patients. In R. P. Cabaj & T. S. Stein (Eds.), *Textbook of homosexuality and mental health* (pp. 897-916). Washington, DC: American Psychiatric Press.

Brown, R. (1973). *Rubyfruit jungle.* New York: Daughters.

Browning, C., Reynolds, A. L., & Dworkin, S. H. (1991). Affirmative psychotherapy for lesbian women. *Counseling Psychologist, 19,* 177-196.

Bryant, S., & Demian. (1994). Relationship characteristics of American gay and lesbian couples: Findings from a national survey. *Journal of Gay & Lesbian Social Services, 1,* 101-117.

Bryant, S., & Demian. (1998). Terms of same-sex endearment. *Siecus Report, 26,* 10-13.

Buhrke, R., & Douce, L. (1991). Training issues for counseling psychologists in working with lesbian women and gay men. *Counseling Psychologist, 19,* 216-234.

Bullough, B., & Bullough, V. (1997). Are transvestites necessarily heterosexual? *Archives of Sexual Behavior, 26,* 1-12.

Bullough, V. L. (1994a). Foreword. In D. Denny (Ed.), *Gender dysphoria: A guide to research* (pp. xv-xix). New York: Garland.

Bullough, V. L. (1994b). *Science in the bedroom: A history of sex research.* New York: Basic Books.

Bullough, V. L. (1998). Alfred Kinsey and the Kinsey report: Historical overview and lasting contributions. *Journal of Sex Research, 35,* 127-131.

Bumpass, L. L., & Aquilino, W. S. (1995). *A social map of midlife: Family and work over the middle life course.* Vero Beach, FL: The MacArthur Foundation Research Network on Successful Midlife Development.

Bumpass, L. L., & Sweet, J. (1989). National estimates of cohabitation: Cohort levels and union stability. *Demography, 26,* 615-625.

Burch, B. (1997). *Other women: Lesbian/bisexual experience and psychoanalytic views of women.* New York: Columbia University Press.

Butler, S. S., & Hope, B. (1999). Health and well-being for late middle-aged and old lesbians in a rural area. *Journal of Gay & Lesbian Social Services, 9,* 27-46.

Buxton, A. P. (1994). *The other side of the closet: The coming-out crisis for straight spouses and families.* New York: John Wiley and Sons.

Cabaj, R. P. (1988). Homosexuality and neurosis: Considerations for psychotherapy. *Journal of Homosexuality, 15,* 13-23.

Cabaj, R. P., & Klinger, R. L. (1996). Psychotherapeutic interventions with lesbian and gay couples. In R. P. Cabaj & T. S. Stein (Eds.), *Textbook of homosexuality and mental health* (pp. 485-502). Washington, DC: American Psychiatric Press.

Cahill, S., South, K., & Spade, J. (2000). *Outing age: Public policy issues affecting gay, lesbian, bisexual, and transgender elders.* New York: The Policy Institute of the National Gay and Lesbian Task Force.

Cain, R. (1991). Relational contexts and information management among gay men. *Families in Society, 72,* 344-352.

Cantu, H. (2003, July 8). Gays saying "I do" to matrimony. *The Dallas Morning News,* pp. A-1, A-10.

Carballo-Diéguez, A. (1989). Hispanic culture, gay male culture, and AIDS: Counseling implications. *Journal of Counseling and Development, 68,* 26-30.

Carroll, L., & Gilroy, P. J. (2002). Transgender issues in counselor preparation. *Counselor Education and Supervision, 3,* 233-242.

Cass, V. C. (1979). Homosexual identity formation: A theoretical model. *Journal of Homosexuality, 4,* 219-235.

Cass, V. C. (1984). Homosexual identity formation: Testing a theoretical model. *Journal of Sex Research, 20,* 143-167.

Cass, V. C. (1996). Sexual orientation identity formation: A western phenomenon. In R. P. Cabaj & T. S. Stein (Eds.), *Textbook of homosexuality and mental health* (pp. 227-251). Washington, DC: American Psychiatric Press.

Chambers, D. (1998). Lesbian divorce: A commentary on legal issues. *American Journal of Orthopsychiatry, 68,* 420-423.

Chan, C. S. (1989). Issues of identity development among Asian-American lesbians and gay men. *Journal of Counseling and Development, 68,* 16-20.

Chan, C. S. (1992). Cultural considerations in counseling Asian American lesbians and gay men. In S. Dworkin & F. Gutiérrez (Eds.), *Counseling gay men and lesbians* (pp. 115-124). Alexandria, VA: American Association for Counseling and Development.

Chan, C. S. (1997). Don't ask, don't tell, don't know: The formation of a homosexual identity and sexual expression among Asian American lesbians. In B. Greene (Ed.), *Ethnic and cultural diversity among lesbians and gay men* (pp. 240-248). Thousand Oaks, CA: Sage Publications.

Chapman, B. E., & Brannock, J. C. (1987). Proposed model of lesbian identity development: An empirical examination. *Journal of Homosexuality, 14,* 69-80.

Charbonneau, D., & Lander, P. (1991). Redefining sexuality: Women becoming lesbian in midlife. In B. Sang, J. Warshow, and A. Smith (Eds.), *Lesbians at midlife: The creative transition* (pp. 35-43). San Francisco: Spinsters.

Chase, C. (2002). "Cultural practice" or "reconstructive surgery"? U.S. genital cutting, the intersex movement, and medical double standards. In S. M. James & C. C. Robertson (Eds.), *Genital cutting and transnational sisterhood: Disputing U.S. polemics* (pp. 126-151). Champaign: University of Illinois Press.

Chernin, J. N., & Johnson, M. R. (2003). *Affirmative psychotherapy and counseling for lesbians and gay men.* Thousand Oaks, CA: Sage Publications.

Claes, J. A., & Moore, W. R. (2000). Issues confronting lesbian and gay elderly: The challenge for health and human services providers. *Journal of Health and Human Services Administration, 23,* 181-202.

Clausen, J. A. (1986). *The life course: A sociological perspective.* Englewood Cliffs, NJ: Prentice-Hall.

Clunis, D. M., & Green, G. D. (2000). *Lesbian couples: A guide to creating healthy relationships.* Seattle, WA: Seal Press.

Clunis, D. M., & Green, G. D. (2003). *The lesbian parenting book: A guide to creating families and raising children,* (Second ed.) New York: Seal Press.

Cochran, S. D., & Mays, V. M. (1988). Disclosure of sexual preference to physicians by black lesbian and bisexual women. *Western Journal of Medicine, 149,* 616-618.

Cohen, K. M., & Savin-Williams, R. C. (1996). Developmental perspectives on coming out to self and others. In R. C. Savin-Williams & K. M. Cohen (Eds.), *The lives of lesbians, gays, and bisexuals: Children to adults* (pp. 113-151). Ft. Worth, TX: Harcourt Brace.

Cohler, B. J. (1982). Personal narrative and the life course. In P. G. Baltes & O. G. Brim (Eds.), *Life-span development and behavior* (pp. 205-241). New York: Academic Press.

Cohler, B., & Boxer, A. (1984). Middle adulthood: Settling into the world—Persons, time, and context. In D. Offer & M. Salbshin (Eds.), *Normality and the lifecycle* (pp. 145-204). New York: Basic Books.

Cohler, B. J. & Galatzer, A. (2000). The course of gay and lesbian lives: Social and psychoanalytic perspectives. Chicago: University of Chicago Press.

Cohler, B. J., & Hostetler, A. J. (2002). Aging, intimate relationships, and life story among gay men. In R. S. Weiss & S. A. Bass (Eds.), *Challenges of the third age: Meaning and purpose in later life* (pp. 137-160). Oxford, England: Oxford University Press.

Cohler, B. J., Hostetler, A. J., & Boxer, A. M. (1998). Generativity, social context, and lived experience: Narratives of gay men in middle adulthood. In D. P. McAdams & E. de St. Aubin (Eds.), *Generativity and adult development* (pp. 265-309). Washington, DC: American Psychological Association.

Cole, E., & Rothblum, E. D. (1990). Commentary on "sexuality and the midlife woman." *Psychology of Women Quarterly, 14,* 509-512.

Cole, E., & Rothblum, E. D. (1991). Lesbian sex at menopause: As good as or better than ever. In B. Sang, J. Warshow, & A. Smith (Eds.), *Lesbians at midlife: The creative transition* (pp. 184-193). San Francisco: Spinsters.

Cole, S. S., Denny, D., Eyler, A. E., and Samons, S. L. (2000). Issues of transgender. In L. T. Szuchman & F. Muscarella (Eds.), *Psychological perspectives on human sexuality* (pp. 149-195). New York: John Wiley and Sons.

Coleman, E. (1985a). Bisexual women in marriages: Conflicts and resolutions in therapy. *Journal of Homosexuality, 11,* 87-99.

Coleman, E. (1985b). Integration of male bisexuality and marriage. *Journal of Homosexuality, 11,* 189-207.

Coleman, E. (1987). Assessment of sexual orientation. *Journal of Homosexuality, 14,* 9-24.

Comstock, G. D. (1991). *Violence against lesbians and gay men.* New York: Columbia University.

Connolly, L. (1996). Long-term care and hospice: The special needs of older gay men and lesbians. *Journal of Gay & Lesbian Social Services, 5,* 77-91.

Conrad, S., & Wincze, J. (1976). Orgasmic reconditioning: A controlled study of the effects upon the sexual arousal and behavior of male homosexuals. *Behavior Therapy, 7,* 155-166.

Coombs, M. (1998). Sexual disorientation: Transgendered people and same-sex marriage. *UCLA Women's Law Journal, 8,* 217-266.

Copper, B. (1988). *Over the hill: Reflections on ageism between women.* Freedom, CA: Crossing.

Coss, C. (1991). Single lesbians speak out. In B. Sang, J. Warshow, & A. Smith (Eds.), *Lesbians at midlife: The creative transition* (pp. 132-140). San Francisco: Spinsters.

Cramer, D. (1986). Gay parents and their children: A review of research and practical implications. *Journal of Counseling and Development, 64,* 504-507.

Cramer, D. W., & Roach, A. J. (1988). Coming out to mom and dad: A study of gay males and their relationships with their parents. *Journal of Homosexuality, 15,* 79-91.

Cramer, E. P. (1997). Strategies for reducing social work students' homophobia. In J. T. Sears & W. L. Williams (Eds.), *Overcoming heterosexism and homophobia: Strategies that work* (pp. 287-298). New York: Columbia University Press.

Crawford, S. (1987). Lesbian families: Psychosocial stress and the family-building process. In Boston Lesbian Psychologies Collective (Eds.), *Lesbian psychologies: Explorations and challenges* (pp. 195-214). Urbana: University of Illinois Press.

Crisp, D., Priest, B., & Torgerson, A. (1998). African American gay men: Developmental issues, choices, and self-concept. *Family Therapy, 25,* 161-168.

Croom, G. L. (2000). Lesbian, gay, and bisexual people of color: A challenge to representative sampling in empirical research. In B. Greene & G. L. Croom (Eds.), *Education, research, and practice in lesbian, gay, bisexual, and transgendered psychology: A resource manual* (Vol. 5) (pp. 263-281). Thousand Oaks, CA: Sage Publications.

Cross, P. & Brookdale Center on Aging—Hunter College (1999). Housing for elderly and lesbians in New York City. Available online at <agingstate.ny.us/explore/project2015/brieflesb.pdf>.

Croteau, J. M., & Morgan, S. (1989). Combating homophobia in AIDS education. *Journal of Counseling and Development, 68,* 86-97.

Croteau, J. M., & Theil, M. J. (1994). Facing gay issues in counseling. *Education Digest, 59,* 25-28.

Croteau, J. M., & von Destinon, M. (1994). A national survey of job search experiences of lesbian, gay and bisexual student affairs professionals. *Journal of College Student Development, 35,* 40-45.

Cruikshank, M. (1992). *The gay and lesbian liberation movement.* New York: Routledge.

Cummerton, J. (1982). Homophobia and social work practice with lesbians. In A. Weick & S. T. Vandiver (Eds.), *Women, power and change* (pp. 104-113). Washington, DC: National Association of Social Workers.

Curran, D., & Parr, D. (1957). Homosexuality: An analysis of 100 male cases. *British Medical Journal, 1,* 797-801.

Dank, B. (1971). Coming out in the gay world. *Psychiatry, 34,* 180-197.

D'Augelli, A. R. (1989). The development of a helping community for lesbians and gay men: A case study in community psychology. *Journal of Community Psychology, 17,* 18-29.

D'Augellli, A. R., Collins, C., Hart, M. (1987). Social support patterns of lesbian women ia a rural helping network. *Journal of Rural Community Psychology, 8,* 12-22.

D'Augelli, A. R., & Garnets, L. D. (1995). Lesbian, gay, and bisexual communities. In A. R. D'Augelli and C. J. Patterson (Eds.), *Lesbians, gay, and bisexual identities over the lifespan* (pp. 293-320). New York: Oxford University Press.

D'Augelli, A. R., & Grossman, A. H. (2001). Disclosure of sexual orientation, victimization, and mental health among lesbian, gay, and bisexual older adults. *Journal of Interpersonal Violence, 16,* 1008-1027.

D'Augelli, A. R., Grossman, A. H., Hershberger, S. L., & O'Connell, T. S. (2001). Aspects of mental health among older lesbian, gay, and bisexual adults. *Aging and Mental Health, 5,* 149-158.

D'Aguelli, A. & Hershberger, S. (1993). Lesbian gay, and bisexual youth in community settings: Personal challeges and mental health problems. *American Journal of Community Psychology, 21,* 421-448.

Davis, D., & Kennedy, E. L. (1986). Oral history and the study of sexuality in the lesbian community: Buffalo, New York, 1940-1960. *Feminist Studies, 12,* 7-26.

Dawson, K. (1982, November). Serving the older gay community. *Siecus Report, 17,* 5-6.

de Monteflores, C., & Schultz. S. (1978). Coming out: Similarities and differences for lesbians and gay men. *Journal of Social Issues, 34,* 59-72.

Deacon, S. A., Reinke, L., & Viers, D. (1998). Cognitive-behavioral therapy for bisexual couples: Expanding the realms of therapy. *American Journal of Family Therapy, 24,* 242-258.

Dean, L., Meyer, I. H., & Robinson, K. (2000, January). *Lesbian, gay, and trans-gendered health: Findings and concerns.* Conference report, Center for Lesbian, Gay, Bisexual, and Transgender Health. New York, pp. 26-31.

Dean, L., Wu, S., & Martin, J. L. (1992). Trends in violence and discrimination against gay men in New York City: 1984-1990. In G. M. Herek & K. T. Berrill (Eds.), *Hate Crimes: Confronting violence against lesbians and gay men* (pp. 46-64). Newbury Park, CA: Sage Publications.

Deevey, S. (1990). Older lesbian women: An invisible minority. *Journal of Gerontological Nursing, 16,* 35-37, 39.

Deevey, S. (1993). Lesbian self-disclosure: Strategies for success. *Journal of Psychosocial Nursing, 31,* 21-26.

Degges-White, S., Rice, B., & Myers, J. E. (2000). Revisiting Cass' theory of sexual identity formation: A study of lesbian development. *Journal of Mental Health Counseling, 22,* 318-333.

D'Emilio, J. (1983). *Sexual politics, sexual communities: The making of a homosexual minority in the United States, 1940-1970.* Chicago: University of Chicago.

D'Emilio, J. (1993). Gay politics and community in San Francisco since World War II. In L. D. Garnets & D. C. Kimmel (Eds.) Psychological perspectives on lesbian & gay male experiences (pp. 59-79). New York: Columbia University Press.

Denny, D. (1997). Transgender: Some historical, cross-cultural, and contemporary models and methods of coping and treatment. In B. Bullough, V. L. Bullough, & J. Elias (Eds.), *Gender blending* (pp. 33-47). Amherst, NY: Prometheus Books.

Denny, D. (1999). Transgender in the United States: A brief discussion. *Siecus Report, 28,* 8-13.

Denny, D. (2002). A selective bibliography of transsexualism. *Journal of Gay & Lesbian Psychotherapy, 6,* 35-66.

Devor, H. (2002). Who are "we"? Where sexual orientation meets gender identity. *Journal of Gay & Lesbian Psychotherapy, 6,* 5-21.

Diamond, L. M. (1996). Attraction and identity: Evidence for sexual fluidity among young lesbian, bisexual, and heterosexual women. Unpublished master's thesis, Cornell University, Ithaca, NY.

Diamond, L. M. (1998). Development of sexual orientation among adolescent and young adult women. *Developmental Psychology, 34,* 1085-1095.

Diamond, M. (2002). Sex and gender are different: Sexual identity and gender identity are different. *Clinical Child Psychology and Psychiatry, 7,* 320-334.

Diamond, M. (2003). Was it a phase? Young women's relinquishment of lesbian/bisexual identities over a 5-year period. *Journal of Personality and Social Psychology, 84,* 352-364.

Diamond, M., & Sigmundson, H. K. (1997a). Management of intersexuality: Guidelines for dealing with persons with ambiguous genitalia. *Archives of Pediatrics and Adolescent Medicine, 151,* 1046-1050.

Diamond, M., & Sigmundson, H. K. (1997b). Sex reassignment at birth: A case report with long-term follow up and clinical implications. *Archives of Pediatric and Adolescent Medicine, 151,* 298-304.

DiAngelo, R. (1997). Heterosexism: Addressing internalized dominance. *Journal of Progressive Human Services, 8,* 5-21.

DiPlacido, J. (1998). Minority stress among lesbians, gay men, and bisexuals: A consequence of heterosexism, homophobia, and stigmatization. In G. M. Herek (Ed.), *Stigma and sexual orientation: Understanding prejudice against lesbians, gay men, and bisexuals* (pp. 138-159). Thousand Oaks, CA: Sage Publications.

Donaldson, C. (2000). Midlife lesbian parenting. *Journal of Gay & Lesbian Social Services, 11,* 119-138.

Donaldson, S. M. (1998). Counselor bias in working with gay men and lesbians: A commentary on Barret and Barzan (1996). *Counseling and Values, 42,* 88-91.

Donovan, J. M. (1992). Homosexual, gay, and lesbian: Defining the words and sampling the populations. In H. L. Minton (Ed.), *Gay and lesbian studies* (pp. 27-47). Binghamton, NY: The Haworth Press.

Dorfman, R., Walters, K., Burke, P., Hardin, L., Karanik, T., Raphael, J., & Silverstein, E. (1995). Old, sad and alone: The myth of the aging homosexual. *Journal of Gerontological Social Work, 24,* 29-44.

Downey, J. I., & Friedman, R. C. (1996). The negative therapeutic reaction and self-hatred in gay and lesbian patients. In R. P. Cabaj & T. S. Stein (Eds.), *Textbook of homosexuality and mental health* (pp. 471-484). Washington, DC: American Psychiatric Press.

Drescher, J. (1998). Contemporary psychoanalytic psychotherapy with gay men: With a commentary on reparative therapy of homosexuality. *Journal of Gay & Lesbian Psychotherapy, 2,* 51-74.

Dubé, E. M. (1997). Sexual identity and intimacy development among two cohorts of sexual minority men. Unpublished master's thesis, Cornell University, Ithaca, NY.

Duberman, M. (1993). *Stonewall.* New York: Dutton.

Dunker, B. (1987). Aging lesbians: Observations and speculations. In Boston Lesbian Psychologies Collective (Eds.), *Lesbian psychologies: Explorations and challenges* (pp. 72-82). Urbana: University of Illinois Press.

Dynes, W. R., & Donaldson, S. (1992). General introduction. In W. R. Dynes & S. Donaldson (Eds.), *Homosexuality and psychology, psychiatry, and counseling* (pp. v-xx). New York: Garland.

Edwards, D. J. (2001, August). Outing the issue. *Nursing Homes: Long Term Care Management, 50,* 40-45. Available at <http://www.nursinghomesmagazine. com/Past Issues.htm?ID=387>.

Ehrenberg, M. (1996). Aging and mental health: Issues in the gay and lesbian community. In C. J. Alexander (Ed.), *Gay and lesbian mental health: A sourcebook for practitioners* (pp. 189-209). Binghamton, NY: Harrington Park Press.

Eldridge, N. S. (1987). Gender issues in counseling same-sex couples. *Professional Psychology: Research and Practice, 18,* 567-572.

Eldridge, N. S., & Barnett, D. C. (1991). Counseling gay and lesbian students. In N. J. Evans & V. A. Walls (Eds.), *Beyond tolerance: Gays, lesbians, and bisexuals on campus* (pp. 147-178). Alexandria, VA: American College Personnel Association.

Ellis, A. L., & Mitchell, R. W. (2000). Sexual orientation. In L. T. Szuchman & F. Muscarella (Eds.), *Psychological perspectives on human sexuality* (pp. 196-231). New York: John Wiley and Sons.

Emerson, S., & Rosenfeld, C. (1996). Stages of adjustment in family members of transgender individuals. *Journal of Family Psychotherapy, 7,* 1-12.

Erikson, E. H. (1980). *Identity and the life cycle.* New York: Norton.

Erikson, E. H. (1982). *The life cycle completed: A review.* New York: Norton.

Espin, O. M. (1984). Cultural and historical influences on sexuality in Hispanic/Latin women: Implications for psychotherapy. In. C. Vance (Ed.), *Pleasure and danger: Exploring female sexuality* (pp. 149-163). London: Routledge & Kegan Paul.

Espin, O. M. (1987). Issues of identity in the psychology of Latina lesbians. In Boston Lesbian Psychologies Collective (Eds.), *Lesbian psychologies: Explorations and challenges* (pp. 35-51). Urbana: University of Illinois Press.

Esterberg, K. G. (1994). Being a lesbian and being in love: Constructing identity through relationships. *Journal of Gay & Lesbian Social Services, 1,* 57-82.

Esterberg, K. G. (1996). Gay cultures, gay communities: The social organization of lesbians, gay men, and bisexuals. In R. C. Savin-Williams & K. M. Cohen (Eds.), *The lives of lesbians, gay men, and bisexuals: Children to adults* (pp. 377-391). Ft. Worth, TX: Harcourt Brace.

Esterberg, K. G. (1997). *Lesbian and bisexual identities: Constructing communities, constructing selves.* Philadelphia: Temple University Press.

Faderman, L. (1981). *Surpassing the love of men: Romantic friendship and love between women from the Renaissance to the present.* New York: Morrow.

Faderman, L. (1991). *Odd girls and twilight lovers: A history of lesbian life in twentieth-century America.* New York: Penguin.

Faderman, L. (1992). The return of butch and femme: A phenomenon in lesbian sexuality of the 1980s and 1990s. *Journal of the History of Sexuality, 2,* 578-596.

Falk, P. J. (1989). Lesbian mothers: Psychosocial assumptions in family law. *American Psychologist, 44,* 941-947.

Faria, G. (1997). The challenge of health care social work with gay men and lesbians. *Social Work in Health Care, 25,* 65-72.

Fassinger, R. E. (1991). The hidden minority: Issues and challenges in working with lesbians and gay men. *Counseling Psychologist, 19,* 157-176.

Fassinger, R. E. (1994, February). *Sexual orientation and identity development: Human dignity for all?* Invited address at the 20th annual Maryland Student Affairs Conference, University of Maryland, College Park.

Fassinger, R. E. (1995). From invisibility to integration: Lesbian identity in the workplace. *The Career Development Quarterly, 44,* 148-166.

Fassinger, R. E. (1996). Notes from the margins: Integrating lesbian experience into the vocational psychology of women. *Journal of Vocational Behavior, 48,* 160-175.

Fassinger, R. E. (1997). Issues in group work with older lesbians. *Group, 21,* 191-210.

Fassinger, R. E., & Miller, B. A. (1996). Validation of an inclusive model of sexual minority identity formation on a sample of gay men. *Journal of Heterosexuality, 32,* 53-78.

Feinberg, L. (1996). *Transgender warriors: Making history from Joan of Arc to RuPaul.* Boston: Beacon Press.

Feldman, M. (1994). Sex, AIDS, and the elderly. *Archives of Internal Medicine, 154,* 19-20.

Fertitta, S. (1984). Never-married women in the middle years. A comparison of lesbians and heterosexuals. Unpublished doctoral dissertation. Wright University, Los Angeles.

Firestein, B. A. (1996). Bisexuality as paradigm shift: Transforming our disciplines. In B. A. Firestein (Ed.), *Bisexuality: The psychology and politics of an invisible minority* (pp. 263-303). Thousand Oaks, CA: Sage Publications.

Ford, C. S. (1948). Sexual behavior among primitive peoples. In D. P. Geddes & E. Curie (Eds.), *About the Kinsey report: Observations by 11 experts* (pp. 26-38). New York: New American Library.

Ford, C. S., & Beach, F. A. (1951). *Patterns of sexual behavior.* New York: Harper & Row.

Fox, R. C. (1991). Development of a bisexual identity: Understanding the process. In L. Hutchins & L. Ka'ahumanu (Eds.), *Bi any other name: Bisexual people speak out* (pp. 29-36). Boston: Alyson.

Francher, J. S., & Henkin, J. (1973). The menopausal queen: Adjustment to aging and the male homosexual. *American Journal of Orthopsychiatry, 43,* 670-674.

Fredriksen, K. I. (1999). Family caregiving responsibilities among lesbians and gay men. *Social Work, 44,* 142-155.

Freedman, M. (1971). *Homosexuality and psychological functioning.* Belmont, CA: Brooks Cole.

Freud, S. (1949). *Three essays on a theory of sexuality.* London: Imago Publishing Company.

Freund, K. (1977). Should homosexuality arouse therapeutic concern? *Journal of Homosexuality, 2,* 235-249.

Friedman, L. (1997). Rural lesbian mothers and their families. *Journal of Gay & Lesbian Social Services, 7,* 73-82.

Friend, R. A. (1980). GAYging: Adjustment and older gay males. *Alternative Lifestyles, 3,* 231-248.

Friend, R. A. (1987). The individual and social psychology of aging: Clinical implications for lesbians and gay men. *Journal of Homosexuality, 14,* 307-331.

Friend, R. A. (1990). Older lesbian and gay people: Responding to homophobia. *Marriage and Family Review, 14,* 241-263.

Friend, R. A. (1991). Older lesbian and gay people: A theory of successful aging. *Journal of Homosexuality, 20,* 99-118.

Frost, J. C. (1997). Group psychotherapy with the aging gay male: Treatment of choice. *Group, 21,* 267-285.

Fullmer, E. M. (1995). Challenging biases against families of older gays and lesbians. In G. C. Smith, S. S. Tobin, E. A. Robertson, T. Chabo, & P. W. Power (Eds.), *Strengthening aging families: Diversity in practice and policy* (pp. 99-119). Thousand Oaks, CA: Sage Publications.

Fullmer, E. M., Shenk, D., & Eastland, L. J. (1999). Negating identity: A feminist analysis of the social invisibility of older lesbians. *Journal of Women & Aging, 11,* 131-148.

Fygetakis, L. M. (1997). Greek American lesbians: Identity odysseys of honorable good girls. In B. Greene (Ed.), *Ethnic and cultural diversity among lesbians and gay men* (pp. 152-190). Thousand Oaks, CA: Sage Publications.

Gagné, P., & Tewksbury, J. R. (1999). Knowledge and power, body and self: An analysis of knowledge systems and the transgendered self. *Sociological Quarterly, 40,* 59-83.

Gagné, P., Tewksbury, R., & McGaughey, D. (1997). Coming out and crossing over: Identity formation and proclamation in a transgender community. *Gender & Society, 11,* 478-508.

Gainor, K. A. (1999). Including transgender issues in lesbian, gay and bisexual psychology: Implications for clinical practice and training. In B. Greene & G. L. Croom (Eds.), *Psychological perspectives on lesbian and gay lives* (Vol. 5) (pp. 131-160). Thousand Oaks, CA: Sage Publications.

Garbo, J. (2000). Transgenders and transsexuals have poor access to healthcare. Available online at <www.gayhealth.com/templates/100351812071520996093 600005/news?record=148>.

Garnets, L. D., Hancock, K. A., Cochran, S. D., Goodchilds, J., & Peplau, L. A. (1991). Issues in psychotherapy with lesbians and gay men: A survey of psychologists. *American Psychologist, 46,* 964-972.

Gartrell, N. (1984). Combating homophobia in the psychotherapy of lesbians. *Women & Therapy, 3,* 13-29.

Gartrell, N., Banks, A., Hamilton, J., Reed, N., Bishop, H., & Rodas, C. (1999). The national lesbian family study. *American Journal of Orthopsychiatry, 69,* 362-369.

GenderPAC (1998). *First National Study on Transviolence.* Waltham, MA: Author.

Gewirtzman, D., & Kaelber, T. (2000). Long-term care issues for the LGBT communities. Presentation given at the Senior Action in a Gay Environment "Out of the Closet—Into the Future: Midlife and Aging in Gay America." Conference New York, May 5-6.

Glassgold, J. M. (1995). Psychoanalysis with lesbians: Self-reflection and agency. In J. Glassgold & S. Iasenza (Eds.), *Lesbians and psychoanalysis: Revolutions in theory and practice* (pp. 203-228). New York: Simon & Schuster.

Gochros, J. S. (1985). Wives' reactions to learning that their husbands are bisexual. *Journal of Homosexuality, 11,* 101-113.

Gochros, J. S. (1989). *When husbands come out of the closet.* Binghamton, NY: The Haworth Press.

Goffman, E. (1963). *Stigma: Notes on the management of spoiled identity.* Englewood Cliffs, NJ: Prentice-Hall.

Golden, C. (1987). Diversity and variability in women's sexual identities. In Boston Lesbian Psychologies Collective (Eds.), *Lesbian psychologies: Explorations and challenges* (pp. 19-34). Urbana: University of Illinois Press.

Golden, C. (1996). What's in a name? Sexual self-identification among women. In R. C. Savin-Williams & K. M. Cohen (Eds.), *The lives of lesbians, gays, and bisexuals: Children to adults* (pp. 229-249). Ft. Worth, TX: Harcourt Brace.

Golombok, S. (2000). Parents' sexual orientation: Heterosexual or homosexual? In S. Golombok (Ed.), *Parenting: What really counts?* (pp. 45-60). Philadelphia: Routledge.

Golombok, S., Spencer, A., & Rutter, M. (1983). Children in lesbian and single-parent households: Psychosexual and psychiatric appraisal. *Journal of Child Psychology, 24,* 551-572.

Gonsiorek, J. C. (1982a). Introduction to mental health issues and homosexuality. *American Behavioral Scientist, 25,* 267-383.

Gonsiorek, J. C. (1982b). Results of psychological testing on homosexual populations. *American Behavioral Scientist, 25,* 385-396.

Gonsiorek, J. C. (1993). Threat, stress, and adjustment: Mental health and the workplace for gay and lesbian individuals. In L. Diamant (Ed.), *Homosexual issues in the workplace* (pp. 242-263). Washington, DC: Taylor & Francis.

Gonsiorek, J. C. (1995). Gay male identities: Concepts and issues. In A. R. D'Augelli & C. J. Patterson (Eds.), *Lesbian, gay, and bisexual identities over the lifespan: Psychological perspectives* (pp. 24-47). New York: Oxford University Press.

Gonsiorek, J. C. (1996). Mental health and sexual orientation. In R. C. Savin-Williams & K. M. Cohen (Eds.), *The lives of lesbians, gay men, and bisexuals: Children to adults* (pp. 462-478). Ft. Worth, TX: Harcourt Brace.

Gonsiorek, J. C., & Weinrich, J. D. (1991). The definition and scope of sexual orientation. In J. C. Gonsiorek & J. Weinrich (Eds.), *Homosexuality: Research implications for public policy* (pp. 1-12). Newbury Park, CA: Sage Publications.

Gray, H., & Dressel, P. (1985). Alternative interpretations of aging among gay males. *The Gerontologist, 25,* 83-87.

Green, R. (1972). Homosexuality as a mental illness. *International Journal of Psychiatry, 10,* 77-128.

Green, R. (1987). *"Sissy boy syndrome" and the development of homosexuality.* New Haven, CT: Yale University Press.

Green, R.-J. (2003). When therapists do not want their clients to be homosexual: A response to Rosik's article. *Journal of Marital & Family Therapy, 29,* 29-38.

Green, R.-J., Bettinger, M., & Zacks, E. (1996). Are lesbian couples fused and gay male couples disengaged? Questioning gender straight jackets. In J. Laird & R.-J. Green (Eds.), *Lesbians and gays in couples and families* (pp. 185-231). San Francisco: Jossey-Bass.

Greene, B. (1994). Ethnic minority lesbians and gay men: Mental health and treatment issues. *Journal of Consulting and Clinical Psychology, 62,* 243-251.

Greene, B. (1996). Lesbians and gay men of color: The legacy of ethnosexual mythologies in heterosexism. In E. D. Rothblum & L. A. Bond (Eds.), *Preventing heterosexism and homophobia* (pp. 59-70). Thousand Oaks, CA: Sage Publications.

Greene, B. (1997). Ethnic minority lesbians and gay men: Mental health and treatment issues. In B. Greene (Ed.), *Ethnic and cultural diversity among lesbians and gay men* (pp. 216-239). Thousand Oaks, CA: Sage Publications.

Grenwald, M. (1984). The SAGE model for serving older lesbians and gay men. *Journal of Social Work and Human Sexuality, 2,* 53-61.

Grossman, A. H., D'Augelli, A. R., & Hershberger, S. L. (2000). Social support networks of lesbian, gay, and bisexual adults 60 years of age and older. *Journal of Gerontology B: Psychology and Social Science, 55,* 171-179.

Grossman, A. H., D'Augelli, A. R., & O'Connell, T. S. (2001). Being lesbian, gay, bisexual, and 60 or older in North America. *Journal of Gay and Lesbian Social Services, 13,* 23-40.

Groves, P. A., & Ventura, L. A. (1983). The lesbian coming-out process: Therapeutic considerations. *The Personnel and Guidance Journal, 62,* 146-149.

Gruskin, E. P. (1999). *Treating lesbians and bisexual women: Challenges and strategies for health professionals.* Thousand Oaks, CA: Sage Publications.

Guidry, L. L. (1999). Clinical intervention with bisexuals: A contextualized understanding. *Professional Psychology: Research and Practice, 30,* 22-26.

Gundlach, R. H., & Riess, B. F. (1968). Self and sexual identity in the female: A study of female homosexuals. In B. F. Riess (Ed.), *New directions in mental health* (pp. 205-231). New York: Grune & Stratton.

Gurevitch, J. (2000). Filial bereavement: Midlife lesbian daughters and intersubjective thoughts. *Journal of Gay & Lesbian Social Services, 11,* 49-76.

Haan, N. (1989). Personality at midlife. In S. Hunter & M. Sundel (Eds.), *Midlife myths: Issues, findings, and practice implications* (pp. 145-156). Newbury Park, CA: Sage Publications.

Haas, S. M., & Stafford, L. (1998). An initial examination of maintenance behaviors in gay and lesbian relationships. *Journal of Social and Personal Relationships, 15,* 846-855.

Haldeman, D. C. (1994). The practice and ethics of sexual orientation conversion therapy. *Journal of Consulting and Clinical Psychology, 62,* 221-227.

Hall, A. S., & Fradkin, H. R. (1992). Affirming gay men's mental health: Counseling with a new attitude. *Journal of Mental Health Counseling, 14,* 362-374.

Hall, M. (1989). Private experiences in the public domain: Lesbians in organizations. In J. Hearn, D. L. Sheppard, P. Tancred-Sheriff, & G. Burrell (Eds.), *The sexuality of organizations* (pp. 125-138). Newbury Park, CA: Sage Publications.

Hall, M., & Gregory, A. (1991). Subtle balances: Love and work in lesbian relationships. In B. Sang, J. Warshow, & A. Smith (Eds.), *Lesbians at midlife: The creative transition* (pp. 122-133). San Francisco: Spinsters.

Hamburger, L. J. (1997). The wisdom of non-heterosexually based senior housing and related services. *Journal of Gay & Lesbian Social Services, 10,* 79-95.

Hancock, K. A. (1995). Psychotherapy with lesbians and gay men. In A. R. D'Augelli & C. J. Patterson (Eds.), *Lesbian, gay, and bisexual identities over the lifespan* (pp. 398-432). New York: Oxford University Press.

Hanscombe, G. E., & Forster, J. (1982). *Rocking the cradle: Lesbian mothers: A challenge in family living.* Boston: Alyson.

Hargaden, H., & Llewellin, S. (1996). Lesbian and gay parenting issues. In D. Davies & C. Neal (Eds.), *Pink therapy: A guide for counselors and therapists working with LGB clients* (pp. 116-130). Philadelphia: Open University Press.

Harrison, A. (1996). Primary care of lesbian and gay patients: Educating ourselves and our students. *Family Medicine, 28,* 10-23.

Harry, J. (1982). Decision making and age differences among gay couples. *Journal of Homosexuality, 8,* 9-21.

Harry, J. (1984). *Gay couples.* New York: Praeger.

Harry, J. (1990). A probability sample of gay males. *Journal of Homosexuality, 19,* 89-104.

Harry, J. (1993). Being out: A general model. *Journal of Homosexuality, 26,* 25-39.

Harry, J., & DeVall, W. B. (1978). *The social organization of gay males.* New York: Praeger.

Harry Benjamin International Gender Dysphoria Association Inc. (1998). The Standards of Care, for gender identity disorders (fifth version). Available online <http://www.tc.umn.edu/~colemoo1/hblyda/hstndrd.htm>.

Hartman, A. (1996). Social policy as a context for lesbian and gay families: The political is personal. In J. Laird & R. J. Green (Eds.), *Lesbians and gays in couples and families* (pp. 69-85). San Francisco: Jossey-Bass.

Hartman, A., & Laird, J. (1998). Moral and ethical issues in working with lesbians and gay men. *Families in Society: Journal of Contemporary Human Services, 79,* 163-276.

Havighurst, R., Neugarten, B., & Tobin, S. (1961). The measurement of life satisfaction. *Journal of Gerontology, 16,* 134-143.

Hayward, R. & Weissfeld, J. (1993). Coming to terms with the era of AIDS: Attitudes of physicians in U.S. residency programs. *Journal of General Internal Medicine, 3,* 10-18.

Healy, T. (1993). A struggle for language: Patterns of self-disclosure in lesbian couples. *Smith College Studies in Social Work, 63,* 247-263.

Henry, G. (1941). *Sex variants: A study of homosexual patterns.* New York: Harpers.

Herdt, G. (1997). *Same sex, different cultures.* Boulder, CO: Westview Press.

Herdt, G., & Beeler, J. (1998). Older gay men and lesbians in families. In C. J. Patterson & A. R. D'Augelli (Eds.), *Lesbian, gay, and bisexual identities in families: Psychological perspectives* (pp. 345-373). New York: Oxford University Press.

Herdt, G. H. (1992). "Coming out" as a rite of passage: A Chicago study. In G. H. Herdt and A. Boxer (Eds.), *Gay culture in America: Essays from the field* (pp. 29-65). Boston: Beacon Press.

Herdt, G. H., Beeler, J., & Rawls, T. W. (1997). Life course diversity among older lesbians and gay men: A study in Chicago. *Journal of Gay, Lesbian, and Bisexual Identity, 2,* 231-246.

Herdt, G. H., & Boxer, A. (1992). Introduction: Culture, history, and life course of gay men. In G. Herdt (Ed.), *Gay culture in America: Essays from the field* (pp. 1-28). Boston: Beacon.

Herdt, G. H., and Boxer, A. (1993). *Children of the horizons: How gay and lesbian teens are leading a way out of the closet.* Boston: Beacon.

Herek, G. M. (1990). The context of anti-gay violence: Notes on cultural and psychological heterosexism. *Journal of Interpersonal Violence, 5,* 316-333.

Herek, G. M. (1991). Myths about sexual orientation: A lawyer's guide to social science research: Law and sexuality. *Review of Lesbian and Gay Legal Issues, 1,* 133-172.

Herek, G. M. (1993). Documenting prejudice against lesbians and gay men on campus: The Yale sexual orientation survey. *Journal of Homosexuality, 25,* 15-30.

Herek, G. M. (1995). Psychological heterosexism in the United States. In A. R. D'Augelli & C. J. Patterson (Eds.), *Lesbian, gay, and bisexual identities over the lifespan: Psychological perspectives* (pp. 321-346). New York: Oxford.

Herek, G. M., Gillis, J. R., and Cogan, J. C. (1999). Psychological sequelae of hate-crime victimization among lesbian, gay, and bisexual adults. *Journal of Consulting and Clinical Psychology, 67,* 945-951.

Hersch, P. (1988, January). Coming of age on city streets. *Psychology Today,* pp. 28-32.

Homosexuals said to face unique midlife issues (1994, July). *Psychiatric News, 29,* 10.

Hooker, E. (1957). The adjustment of the male overt homosexual. *Journal of Projective Techniques, 211,* 18-31.

Hooyman, N. R., & Lustbader, W. (1986). *Taking care: Supporting older people and their families.* New York: Free Press.

Hopcke, R. H. (1992). Midlife, gay men, and the AIDS epidemic. *Quadrant, 25,* 101-109.

Horowitz, J. L., & Newcomb, M. D. (2001). A multidimensional approach to homosexual identity. *Journal of Homosexuality, 42,* 1-19.

Hostetler, A. J. (2000). Lesbian and gay lives across the adult years. In B. J. Cohler & R. M. Galatzer (Eds.), *The course of gay and lesbian lives: Social and psycho-analytic perspectives* (pp. 193-251). Chicago: University of Chicago Press.

Hostetler, A. J., & Cohler, B. J. (1997). Partnership, singlehood, and the lesbian and gay life course: A research agenda. *Journal of Gay, Lesbian, and Bisexual Identity, 2,* 199-230.

Hostetler, A., & Herdt, G. (1998). Culture, sexual lifeways and developmental subjectivities: Rethinking sexual taxonomies. *Social Research, 65,* 249-290.

Hughes, R. B., & Friedman, A. L. (1994, October). AIDS-related ethical and legal issues for mental health professionals. *Journal of Mental Health Counseling, 16,* 445-458.

Human Rights Campaign. (2000). Unique housing challenges. In *Aging: Senior housing.* Available online at <http:/www.hrc.org/>.

Human Rights Campaign. (2004). Domestic partners. Available online at <http://www.hrc.org>.

Humphreys, N. A., & Quam, J. K. (1998). Middle-aged and old gay, lesbian, and bisexual adults. In G. A. Appleby & J. W. Anastas (Eds.), *Not just a passing phase: Social work with gay, lesbian, and bisexual people* (pp. 245-267). New York: Columbia University Press.

Hunt, S., & Main, T. L. (1997). Sexual orientation confusion among spouses of transvestites and transsexuals following disclosure of spouse's gender dysphoria. *Journal of Psychology & Human Sexuality, 9,* 39-52.

Hunter, S. (1994, November). Crisis versus transition: How to assess which one fits your midlife clients. Paper presented at the meeting of the National Association of Social Workers/Texas Annual Conference, Dallas.

Hunter, S., and Hickerson, J. (2003). *Affirmative practice: Understanding and working with Lesbian, gay, bisexual, and transgender persons.* Washington, DC: NASW Press.

Hunter, S., Shannon, C., Knox, J., & J. I. Martin. (1998). *Lesbian, gay, and bisexual youth and adults: Knowledge for human services practice.* Thousand Oaks, CA: Sage Publications.

Hunter, S., Sundel, S., & Sundel, M. (2002). *Women at midlife: Life experiences and implications for the helping professions.* Washington, DC: NASW Press.

Hutchins, L. (1996). Bisexuality: Politics and community. In B. A. Firestein (Ed.), *Bisexuality: The psychology and politics of an invisible minority* (pp. 240-259). Thousand Oaks, CA: Sage Publications.

Icard, L. D. (1996). Assessing the psychosocial well-being of African American gays: A multidimensional perspective. *Journal of Gay & Lesbian Social Services, 5,* 25-49.

Igartua, K. J. (1998). Therapy with lesbian couples: The issues and the interventions. *Canadian Journal of Psychiatry, 43,* 391-396.

Ilnytzky, U. (1999). '98 anti-gay attacks fewer but more violent. *Dallas Voice, 15,* 13-14.

Isay, R. A. (1990). Psychoanalytic theory and the therapy of gay men. In D. P. McWhirter, S. A. Sanders, & J. M. Reinisch (Eds.), *Homosexuality/heterosexuality: Concepts of sexual orientation* (pp. 283-303). New York: Oxford University Press.

Isay, R. A. (1996). *Becoming gay: The journey of self-acceptance.* New York: Pantheon Books.

Israel, G. E., & Tarver, D. E. (1997). *Transgender care: Recommended guidelines, practical information and personal accounts.* Philadelphia: Temple University Press.

Jacobs, M. A., & Brown, L. B. (1997). American Indian lesbians and gays: An exploratory story. *Journal of Gay & Lesbian Social Services, 6,* 29-41.

Jacobs, R. J., Rasmussen, L. A., & Hohman, M. M. (1999). The social support needs of older lesbians, gay men, and bisexuals. *Journal of Gay & Lesbian Social Services, 9,* 1-30.

Jacobson, R., & Wright, J. (1992). Financial planning: Making the best use of your money. In B. Berzon (Ed.), *Positively gay: New approaches to gay and lesbian life* (pp. 183-194). Berkeley, CA: Celestial Arts.

Jacobson, S. (1995). Methodological issues in research on older lesbians. *Journal of Gay & Lesbian Social Services, 3,* 43-56.

Jacobson, S. & Grossman, A. H. (1996). Older lesbians and gay men: Old myths, new images, and future directions. In R. C. Savin-Williams & K. M. Cohen (Eds.), *The lives of lesbians, gay, and bisexuals: Children to adults* (pp. 345-373). Fort Worth, TX: Harcourt, Brace.

James, S. E., & Murphy, B. C. (1998). Gay and lesbian relationships in a changing social context. In C. J. Patterson & A. R. D'Augelli (Eds.), *Lesbian, gay, and bisexual identities in families: Psychological perspectives* (pp. 99-121). New York: Oxford University Press.

Jay, K. & Young, A. (Eds.), (1972). *Out of the closets: Voices of gay liberation.* New York: Douglas/Links.

Jeffreys, S. (1994). The queer disappearance of lesbians: Sexuality in the academy. *Women's Studies International Forum, 17,* 459-472.

Jensen, K. L. (1999). *Lesbian epiphanies: Women coming out in later life.* Binghamton, NY: Harrington Park Press.

Johansson, W. (1990). Law, United States. In W. R. Dynes (Ed.), *Encyclopedia of homosexuality* (pp. 692-698). New York: Garland.

Johnson, B. (1990). Survey reveals male and female differences in sexual behaviors of older adults. *Contemporary Sexuality, 24,* 3.

Johnson, S. M., & O'Connor, E. (2001). *For lesbian parents: Your guide to helping your family grow up happy, healthy, and proud.* New York: Guilford Press.

Jones, B. E. (2001). Is having the luck of growing old in the gay, lesbian, bisexual, transgender community good or bad luck? *Journal of Gay & Lesbian Social Services, 13,* 13-14.

Jones, B. E., & Hill, M. J. (1996). African American lesbians, gay men, and bisexuals. In R. P. Cabaj & T. S. Stein (Eds.), *Textbook of homosexuality and mental health* (pp. 549-561). Washington, DC: American Psychiatric Press.

Jones, M. A., & Gabriel, M. A. (1999). Utilization of psychotherapy by lesbians, gay men, and bisexuals: Findings from a nationwide survey. *American Journal of Orthopsychiatry, 69,* 209-219.

Jones, T. C., & Nystrom, N. M. (2002). Looking back . . . looking forward: Addressing the lives of lesbians 55 and older. *Journal of Women & Aging, 14,* 59-76.

Jones, T. C., Nystrom, N. M., Fredriksen, K. I., Clunis, D. M., & Freeman, P. (1999, March). Looking back . . . Looking forward: Addressing the lives of lesbians 55 and older. Presented at the Annual Program Meeting, Council on Social Work Education, San Francisco, CA.

Jost, K. (2000). Gay-Rights Update. *CQ Researcher, 10,* 307-327.

JSI Research and Training Institute Inc. (2000). *Access to Health care for transgendered persons in Greater Boston.* Boston: Gay, Lesbian, Bisexual, and Transgender Health Access Project.

Kanuha, V. (1990). Compounding the triple jeopardy: Battering in lesbian of color relationships. *Women and Therapy, 9,* 169-184.

Karp, B. (2000). *Let us decide: Healthcare proxies and living wills.* Available online at <www.gayhealth.com>.

Kehoe, M. (1986). Lesbians over 65: A triple invisible minority. *Journal of Homosexuality, 12,* 139-152.

Kehoe, M. (1989). *Lesbians over 60 speak for themselves.* Binghamton, NY: Harrington Park Press.

Kelly, J. (1975). *Brothers and brothers: The gay man's adaptation to aging* (Doctoral dissertation, Brandeis University, 1974). *Dissertation Abstracts International, 36,* 3130 A.

Kelly, J. (1977). The aging male homosexual: Myth and reality. *The Gerontologist, 17,* 328-332.

Kelly, J. (1980). Homosexuality and aging. In J. Marmor (Ed.), *Homosexual behavior: A modern reappraisal* (pp. 176-193). New York: Basic Books.

Kelly, M. (1998). View from the field out in education: Where the personal and political collide. *Siecus Report, 26,* 14-15.

Kennedy, E. L., & Davis, M. D. (1993). *Boots of leather, slippers of gold: The history of a lesbian community.* New York: Routledge.

Kertzner, R. (1999). Self-appraisal of life experience and the psychological adjustment in midlife gay men. *Journal of Psychology and Human Sexuality, 11,* 43-64.

Kertzner, R. M. (2001). The adult life course and homosexual identity in midlife gay men. *Annual Review of Sex Research, 12,* 75-92.

Khayatt, D. (2002). Toward a queer identity. *Sexualities, 5,* 487-501.

Kimmel, D. C. (1977). Psychotherapy and the older gay man. *Psychotherapy: Theory, Research and Practice, 14,* 386-393.

Kimmel, D. C. (1978). Adult development and aging: A gay perspective. *Journal of Social Issues, 34,* 113-130.

Kimmel, D. C. (1979). Adjustments to aging among gay men. In B. Berzon & R. Leighton (Eds.), *Positively gay* (pp. 146-158). Berkeley, CA: Celestial Arts.

Kimmel, D. C. (1979-1980). Life-history interviews of aging gay men. *International Journal of Aging & Human Development, 10,* 239-248.

Kimmel, D. C. (1992). The families of older gay men and lesbians. *Generations, 16,* 37-38.

Kimmel, D. (1993). Adult development and aging: A gay perspective. In L. D. Garnets & D. C. Kimmel (Eds.), *Psychological perspectives on lesbian and gay male experiences* (pp. 517-534). New York: Columbia University Press.

Kimmel, D. C. (2002). Aging and sexual orientation. In B. E. Jones & M. J. Hill (Eds.), *Mental health issues in lesbian, gay, bisexual, and transgender communities* (pp. 17-36). Washington, DC: American Psychiatric Publishing, Inc.

Kimmel, D. C., & Sang, B. E. (1995). Lesbians and gay men in midlife. In A. R. D'Augelli & C. J. Patterson (Eds.), *Lesbian, gay, and bisexual identities over the lifespan: Psychological perspectives* (pp. 190-214). New York: Oxford.

Kinsey, A. C., Pomeroy, W. B., & Martin, C. E. (1948). *Sexual behavior in the human male.* Philadelphia: W. B. Saunders.

Kinsey, A. C., Pomeroy, W. B., Martin, C. E., & Gebbard, P. H. (1953). *Sexual behavior in the human female.* Philadelphia: W. B. Saunders.

Kirkpatrick, M. (1988). Clinical implications of lesbian mother studies. In E. Coleman (Ed.), *Integrated identity for gay men and lesbians: Psychotherapeutic approaches for emotional well-being* (pp. 201-211). Binghamton, NY: Harrington Park Press.

Kirkpatrick, M. (1989a). Lesbians: A different middle-age? In J. Oldham & R. Liebert (Eds.), *New psychoanalytic perspectives: The middle years* (pp. 135-148). New Haven, CT: Yale University.

Kirkpatrick, M. (1989b). Middle age and the lesbian experience. *Women's Studies Quarterly, 1-2,* 87-86.

Kirkpatrick, M., Smith, C., & Roy, R. (1981). Lesbian mothers and their children: A comparative survey. *American Journal of Orthopsychiatry, 51,* 545-551.

Kitzinger, C. (1991). Lesbian and gay men in the workplace: Psychosocial issues. In M. J. Davidson & J. Earnshaw (Eds.), *Vulnerable workers: Psychosocial and legal issues* (pp. 223-257). New York: John Wiley and Sons.

Kitzinger, C., & Coyle, A. (1995). Lesbian and gay couples: Speaking of difference. *Psychologist, 8,* 64-69.

Klein, F. (1993). *The bisexual option* (Second ed.). Binghamton, NY: Harrington Park Press.

Klein, F., Sepekoff, B., & Wolf, T. J. (1985). Sexual orientation: A multi-variable dynamic process. *Journal of Homosexuality, 11,* 35-49.

Kochman, A. (1997). Gay and lesbian elderly: Historical overview and implications for social work practice. *Journal of Gay & Lesbian Social Services, 6,* 1-10.

Kooden, H. (1997). Successful aging in the middle-aged gay man: A contribution to developmental theory. *Journal of Gay & Lesbian Social Services, 6,* 21-43.

Kooden, H., & Flowers, C. (2000). *Golden men: The power of gay midlife.* New York: Avon Books.

Kooperman, L. (1994). A survey of gay and bisexual men age 50 and older: AIDS related knowledge, attitude, belief and behavior. *AIDS Patient Care, 8,* 115-116.

Kravets, D. (2004, August 12). Calif. court voids S.F. gay marriages. Associated Press. Available online at <http://apnews.myway.com/article/20040812/D84DVM900. html>.

Kuehlwein, K. T. (1992). Working with gay men. In A. M. Freeman & F. M. Dattilio (Eds.), *Comprehensive casebook of cognitive therapy* (pp. 249-255). New York: Plenum Press.

Kuehlwein, K. T., & Gottschalk, D. I. (2000). Legal and psychological issues confronting lesbian, bisexual, and gay couples and families. In F. W. Kaslow (Ed.) *Handbook of couples and family forensic: A sourcebook for mental health and legal professionals* (pp. 164-187). New York: John Wiley and Sons.

Kurdek, L. A. (1988a). Perceived social support in gays and lesbians in cohabiting relationships. *Journal of Personality and Social Psychology, 54,* 504-509.

Kurdek, L. A. (1988b). Relationship quality of gay and lesbian cohabiting couples. *Journal of Homosexuality, 15,* 93-118.

Kurdek, L. A. (1994a). Conflict resolution styles in gay, lesbian, heterosexual nonparent, and heterosexual parent couples. *Journal of Marriage and the Family, 56,* 705-722.

Kurdek, L.A. (1994b). The nature and correlates of relationship quality in gay, lesbian, and heterosexual cohabiting couples. In B. Greene & G. Herek (Eds.), *Contemporary perspectives on gay and lesbian psychology: Theory, research, and applications* (pp. 133-155). Beverly Hills, CA: Sage Publications.

Kurdek, L. A. (1995a). Assessing multiple determinants of relationship commitment in cohabitating gay, cohabitating lesbian, dating heterosexual, and married heterosexual couples. *Family Relations, 44,* 261-266.

Kurdek, L. A. (1995b). Developmental changes in relationship quality in gay and lesbian cohabitating couples. *Developmental Psychology, 31,* 86-94.

Kurdek, L. A. (1997). Adjustment to relationship dissolution in gay, lesbian, and heterosexual partners. *Personal Relationships, 4,* 145-161.

Kurdek, L. A., & Schmitt, J. P. (1986a) Interaction of sex role self-concept with relationship quality and relationship beliefs in married, heterosexual cohabiting, gay and lesbian relationships. *Journal of Personality and Social Psychology, 51,* 365-370.

Kurdek, L. A., & Schmitt, J. P. (1986b). Relationship quality of partners in heterosexual married, heterosexual cohabiting, and gay and lesbian relationships. *Journal of Personality and Social Psychology, 51,* 711-720.

Kurdek, L. A., & Schmitt, J. P. (1987). Perceived emotional support from family and friends in members of homosexual, married, and heterosexual cohabiting couples. *Journal of Homosexuality, 14,* 57-68.

Laird, J. (1994). Lesbian families: A cultural perspective. In M. P. Mirkin (Ed.), *Women in context: Toward a feminist reconstruction of psychotherapy* (pp. 118-148). New York: Guilford Press.

Laird, J. (1995). Family-centered practice in the postmodern era. *Families in Society: Journal of Contemporary Human Services, 76,* 150-162.

Laird, J. (1996). Family-centered practice with lesbian and gay families. *Families in Society: Journal of Contemporary Human Services, 77,* 559-572.

Laird, J. (2000). Gender in lesbian relationships: Cultural, feminist, and constructionist reflections. *Journal of Marital and Family Therapy, 26,* 455-467.

Lander, P. S., & Charbonneau, C. (1990). The new lesbian in midlife: Reconstructing sexual identity. In J. Hurtig, K. Gillogly, & T. Gulevich (Eds.), *Gender tranformations, Michigan Discussions in Anthropology, 9,* 1-14.

Laumann, E. D., Gagnon, J. H., Michael, R. T., & Michaels, S. (1994). *The social organization of sexuality: Sexual practices in the United States.* Chicago: University of Chicago Press.

Leaveck, A. (1994). Perceived parental reactions to same-sex sexual orientation disclosure: A search for predictors. Unpublished doctoral dissertation, Central Michigan University, Mount Pleasant.

Lee, J. A. (1977). Going public: A study in the sociology of homosexual liberation. *Journal of Homosexuality, 3,* 49-78.

Lee, J. A. (1987). What can homosexual aging studies contribute to theories of aging? *Journal of Homosexuality, 13,* 43-71.

Lee, J. A. (1989). Invisible men: Canada's aging homosexuals. Can they be assimilated into Canada's "liberated" gay communities? *Canadian Journal on Aging, 8,* 29-43.

Lee, J. A. (1990). Aging. In W. Dynes (Ed.), *Encyclopedia of homosexuality* (pp. 26-29). New York: Garland.

Lelyveld, Nita (2003, October 13). Group seeks housing help for elderly gays. *Los Angeles Times.* Available online at <http://www.hrc.org/Content/ContentGroups/News3/20037/Group_Seeks_Housing_Help_for_Elderly_Gays.htm>.

Lesbian Life (2004a). Where can gays legally marry? Available online at <http://lesbianlife.about.com/cs/wedding/a/wheremarriage.htm>.

Lesbian Life (2004b). The difference between marriage and civil unions. Available online at <http://lesbianlife.about.com/cs/wedding/a/unionvmarriage.htm>.

Levine, J. A., & Altman, C. (2002). Collaborating to support lesbian and gay caregivers for people with Alzheimer's. *Outword, 8,* 7-8.

Levine, M. P. (1992). The life and death of gay clones. In G. Herdt (Ed.), *Gay culture in America: Essays from the field* (pp. 68-86). Boston: Beacon.

Levine, M. P., & Leonard, R. (1984). Discrimination against lesbians in the work force. *Signs, 9,* 700-710.

Levine, S. B., Brown, G. B., Coleman, E., Hage, J. J., Cohen-Kettenis, P., Van Maasdam, J., Petersen, M., Pfafflin, F., & Schaefer, L. (1998, April-June). Harry Benjamin International Gender Dysphoria Association's standards of care for gender identity disorders. *International Journal of Transgenderism, 2,* 2.

Levinger, G. C. (1982). A social exchange view of the dissolution of pair relationships. In F. L. Nye (Ed.), *Family relationships: Rewards and costs* (pp. 97-112). Beverly Hills, CA: Sage Publications.

Levinson, D., Darrow, C. N., Klein, E. B., Levinson, M. H., & McKee, B. (1978). *The seasons of a man's life.* New York: Knopf.

Levy, E. F. (1995). Feminist social work practice with lesbian and gay clients. In N. Van Den Bergh (Ed.), *Feminist practice in the 21st century* (pp. 278-294). Washington, DC: NASW Press.

Lewes, K. (1988). *The psychoanalytic theory of male homosexuality.* New York: Simon & Schuster.

Liddle, B. J. (1996). Therapist sexual orientation, gender, and counseling practices as they relate to ratings of helpfulness by gay and lesbian clients. *Journal of Counseling Psychology, 41,* 394-401.

Liddle, B. J. (1997). Gay and lesbian clients' selection of therapists and utilization of therapy. *Psychotherapy, 34,* 11-18.

Liddle, B. J. (1999). Recent improvement in mental health services to lesbian and gay clients. *Journal of Homosexuality, 37,* 127-137.

Lieberman, M., & Tobin, S. (1983). *The experience of old age: Stress, coping, and survival.* New York: Basic Books.

Linde, R. (1994). Impact of AIDS on adult gay male development: Implications for psychotherapy. In S. A. Cadwell, R. A. Burnhan, & M. Forstein (Eds.), *Therapists on the frontline: Psychotherapy with gay men in the age of AIDS* (pp. 25-31). Washington, DC: American Psychiatric Press.

Linsk, N. L. (1997). Experience of old gay and bisexual men living with HIV/AIDS. *Journal of Gay, Lesbian, and Bisexual Identity, 2,* 285-308.

Liu, P., & Chan, C. C. (1996). Lesbian, gay, and bisexual Asian Americans and their families. In J. Laird & R.-J. Green (Eds.), *Lesbians and gays in couples and families: A handbook for therapists* (pp. 137-152). San Francisco: Jossey-Bass.

Lombardi, E. L. (1999). Integration within a transgender social network and its effect upon members' social and political activity. *Journal of Homosexuality, 37,* 109-126.

Lombardi, E. (2001). Enhancing transgender health scare. *American Journal of Public Health, 91,* 869-872.

Longres, J. F. (2000). *Human behavior and the social environment* (Third ed.). Itasca, IL: F. E. Peacock.

Lopez, R. A., & Lam, B. T. (1998). Social supports among Vietnamese American gay men. *Journal of Gay and Lesbian Social Services, 8,* 29-50.

Lott-Whitehead, L., & Tully, C. T. (1993). The family lives of lesbian mothers. *Smith College Studies in Social Work, 63,* 266-280.

Loughery, J. (1998). *The other side of silence: Men's lives and gay identities: A twentieth-century history.* New York: Henry Holt.

Loulan, J. (1987). *Lesbian passion: Loving ourselves and each other.* San Francisco: Spinsters/Aunt Lute.

Lourea, D. N. (1985). Psycho-social issues related to counseling bisexuals. *Journal of Homosexuality, 11,* 51-62.

Lucco, A. J. (1987). Planned retirement housing preferences of older homosexuals. *Journal of Homosexuality, 14,* 35-56.

Lynch, F. R. (1992). Nonghetto gays: An ethnography of suburban homosexuals. In G. Herdt (Ed.), *Gay culture in America: Essays from the field* (pp. 165-201). Boston: Beacon.

Lynch, J. M., & Reilly, M. E. (1986). Role relationships: Lesbian perspectives. *Journal of Homosexuality, 12,* 53-69.

MacDonald, B. J. (1998). Issues in therapy with gay and lesbian couples. *Journal of Sex & Marital Therapy, 24,* 165-190.

MacDonald, B. & Rich, C. (1983). *Look me in the eye: Old women, aging, and age-ism.* San Francisco: Spinster.

Mackelprang, R. W., Ray, J., & Hernandez-Peck, M. (1996). Social work education and sexual orientation: Faculty, student, and curriculum issues. *Journal of Gay & Lesbian Social Services, 5,* 17-31.

Mail, P. D. (2002). The case for expanding educational and community-based programs that serve lesbian, gay, bisexual, and transgender populations. *Clinical Research and Regulatory Affairs, 19,* 223-273.

Mallon, G. (1998a). Knowledge for practice with gay and lesbian persons. In G. P. Mallon (Ed.), *Foundations of social work practice with lesbian and gay persons* (pp. 1-30). Binghamton, NY: The Haworth Press.

Mallon, G. P. (1998b). Social work practice with gay men and lesbians within families. In G. P. Mallon (Ed.), *Foundations of social work practice with lesbian and gay persons* (pp. 145-180). Binghamton, NY: The Haworth Press.

Malyon, A. K. (1981-1982). Psychotherapeutic implications of internalized homophobia in gay men. *Journal of Homosexuality, 7,* 56-59.

Manalansan IV, M. F. (1996). Double minorities: Latino, black, and Asian men who have sex with men. In R. C. Savin-Williams & K. M. Cohen (Eds.), *The lives of lesbian, gay men, and bisexuals: Children to adults* (pp. 393-425). Ft. Worth, TX: Harcourt Brace.

Mann, W. (1997, May). Gray gays: Aging gay men and lesbians face unique challenges. Available online at <http://www.bostonphoenix.com/archive/1in10/97/05/GRAY_GAYS.html>.

Markowitz, L. M. (1991, January-February). Homosexuality: Are we still in the dark? *Family Therapy Networker,* 26-29, 31-35.

Marks, R. (Ed.). (1993, April). *Focus: A guide to AIDS research and counseling* (Publication of AIDS Health Project, no. 8). San Francisco: University of California.

Marmor, J. (1972). Homosexuality: Mental illness or moral dilemma? *International Journal of Psychiatry, 10,* 114-117.

Marmor, J. (1980). Overview: The multiple roots of homosexual behavior. In J. Marmor (Ed.), *Homosexual behavior: A modern reappraisal* (pp. 3-22). New York: Basic.

Marsiglia, F. F. (1998). Homosexuality and Latinos/as: Toward an integration of identities. *Journal of Gay & Lesbian Social Services, 8,* 113-125.

Martin, A. (1982). Some issues in the treatment of gay and lesbian patients. *Psychotherapy: Theory, Research and Practice, 19,* 341-348.

Martin, A. (1993). *The lesbian and gay parenting handbook.* New York: Harper-Collins.

Martin, A. D. (1982). Learning to hide: Socialization of the gay adolescent. *Adolescent Psychiatry, 10,* 52-64.

Martin, A. D., & Hetrick, E. S. (1988). The stigmatization of the gay and lesbian adolescent. *Journal of Homosexuality, 15,* 163-183.

Martin, D., & Lyon, P. (1992). The older lesbian. In B. Berzon & R. Leighton (Eds.), *Positively gay* (pp. 111-120). Berkeley: Celestial Arts.

Martin, D., & Lyon, P. (1995). Lesbian liberation begins. *The Harvard Lesbian & Gay Review, 2,* 15-18.

Martinez, D. G. (1998). Mujer, Latina, lesbian—Notes on the multidimensionality of economic and sociopolitical injustice. *Journal of Gay & Lesbian Social Services, 8,* 99-112.

Mason-John, V., & Khambatta, A. (1993). *Lesbians talk: Making black waves.* London: Scarlett Press.

Masters, W., & Johnson, V. (1979). *Homosexuality in perspective.* Boston: Little, Brown.

Matteson, D. R. (1987). The heterosexually married gay and lesbian parent. In F. W. Bozett (Ed.), *Gay and lesbian parents* (pp. 138-161). New York: Praeger.

Matteson, D. R. (1995). Counseling with bisexuals. *Individual Psychology, 51,* 144-159.

Matteson, D. R. (1996a). Counseling and psychotherapy with bisexual and exploring clients. In B. A. Firestein (Ed.), *Bisexuality: The psychology and politics of an invisible minority* (pp. 185-213). Thousand Oaks, CA: Sage Publications.

Matteson, D. R. (1996b). Psychotherapy with bisexual individuals. In R. P. Cabaj & T. S. Stein (Eds.), *Textbook of homosexuality and mental health* (pp. 433-449). Washington, DC: American Psychiatric Press.

Matthews, C. R., & Lease, S. H. (2000). Focus on lesbian, gay, and bisexual families. In R. M. Perez, K. A. DeBord, & K. J. Bieschke (Eds.), *Handbook of counseling and psychotherapy with lesbian, gay, and bisexual clients* (pp. 249-273). Washington, DC: American Psychological Association.

Maurer, L. (1999). Transgressing sex and gender: Deconstruction zone ahead? *Siecus Report, 28,* 14-21.

Mayerson, P., & Lief, H. (1965). Psychotherapy of homosexuals: A follow-up study of nineteen cases. In J. Marmor (Ed.), *Sexual inversion* (pp. 302-344). New York: Basic Books.

Mays, V. M., Chatters, L. M., Cochran, S. D., & Mackness, J. (1998). African American families in diversity: Gay men and lesbians as participants in family networks. *Journal of Comparative Family Studies, 29,* 73-87.

McAllan, L. D., & Ditillo, D. (1994). Addressing the needs of lesbian and gay clients with disabilities. *Journal of Applied Rehabilitation Counseling, 25,* 26-35.

McCarn, S. R., & Fassinger, R. E. (1996). Revisioning sexual minority identity formation: A new model of lesbian identity and its implications for counseling and research. *Counseling Psychologists, 24,* 508-534.

McDougall, G. J. (1993). Therapeutic issues with gay and lesbian elders. *Clinical Gerontologist, 14,* 45-57.

McGrath, E. (1990, August). New treatment strategies for women in the middle. Paper presented at the annual convention of the American Psychological Association, Boston.

McHenry, S. S., & Johnson, J. W. (1993). Homophobia in the therapist and gay or lesbian client: Conscious and unconscious illusions in self-hate. *Psychotherapy, 30,* 141-151.

McKenna, W., & Kessler, S. J. (2000). Retrospective response. *Feminism & Psychology, 10,* 66-72.

McVinney, L. D. (1998). Social work practice with gay male couples. In G. P. Mallon (Ed.), *Foundations of social work practice with lesbian and gay persons* (pp. 209-227). Binghamton, NY: The Haworth Press.

McWhirter, D. P., & Mattison, A. M. (1984). *The male couple.* Englewood Cliffs, NJ: Prentice-Hall.

Meris, D. (2001). Responding to the mental health and grief concerns of homeless HIV-infected gay men. *Journal of Gay & Lesbian Social Services, 13,* 103-111.

Messing, A. E., Schoenberg, R., & Stephens, R. K. (1983-1984). Confronting homophobia in health care settings: Guidelines for social work practice. *Journal of Social Work & Human Sexuality, 2,* 65-74.

Meyer I. H. (2001). Why lesbian, gay, bisexual and transgender public health? *American Journal of Public Health, 91,* 857-858.

Miller, N. (1990). *In search of gay America.* New York: Harper & Row.

Minnigerode, F. A. (1976). Age-status labeling in homosexual men. *Journal of Homosexuality, 1,* 273-276.

Minnigerode, F., and Adelman, M. (1976). Adaptations of aging homosexual men and women. Paper presented at the Convention of the Gerontological Society, New York, October.

Minnigerode, F., & Adelman, M. (1978). Elderly homosexual women and men: Report on a pilot study. *Family Cooordinator, 27,* 451-456.

Minnigerode, F. A., Adelman, M. R., & Fox, D. (1980). Aging and homosexuality: Physical and psychological well-being. Unpublished manuscript, University of San Francisco.

Minton, H. L., & McDonald, G. J. (1983-1984). Homosexual identity formation as a developmental process. *Journal of Homosexuality, 9,* 91-104.

Mintz, E. (1996). Overt male homosexuals in combined group and individual treatment. *Journal of Counseling Psychology, 20,* 193-198.

Mitchell, V. (2000). The bloom is on the rose: The impact of midlife on the lesbian couple. *Journal of Gay & Lesbian Social Services, 11,* 33-48.

Mitchell, V., & Helson, R. (1990). Women's prime of life: Is it the 50s? *Psychology of Women Quarterly, 14,* 451-470.

Mock, S. E. (2001). Retirement intentions of same-sex couples. *Journal of Gay & Lesbian Social Services, 13,* 81-86.

Money, J. (1998). Homosexuality: Bipotentiality, terminology, and history. In E. J. Haeberle and R. Gindorf (Eds.), *Bisexualities: The ideology and practice of sexual contact with both men and women* (pp. 118-128). New York: Continuum.

Moore, W. R. (2002). Lesbian and gay elders: Connecting care providers through a telephone support group. *Journal of Gay & Lesbian Social Services, 14,* 23-41.

Morales, E. S. (1992). Counseling Latino gays and Latina lesbians. In S. Dworkin & F. Gutiérrez (Eds.), *Counseling gay men and lesbians: Journey to the end of the rainbow* (pp. 125-139). Alexandria, VA: American Association for Counseling and Development.

Morales, E. S. (1996). Gender roles among Latino gay and bisexual men: Implications for family and couple therapy. In J. Laird & R.-J. Green (Eds.), *Lesbians and gays in couples and families: A handbook for therapists* (pp. 272-297). San Francisco: Jossey-Bass.

Morgan, K. S. (1992). Caucasian lesbians' use of psychotherapy: A matter of attitude? *Psychology of Women Quarterly, 16,* 127-130.

Morin, S. F. (1977). Heterosexual bias in research on lesbianism and male homosexuality. *American Psychologist, 32,* 629-637.

Morin, S. F., & Rothblum, E. D. (1991). Removing the stigma: Fifteen years of progress. *American Psychologist, 46,* 947-949.

Moss, M. S., & Moss, S. Z. (1983-1984). The impact of parental death on middle-aged children. *Omega, 14,* 65-71.

Moss, M. S. & Moss, S. Z. (1989). The death of a parent. In R. A. Kalish (Ed.), *Midlife loss: Coping strategies* (pp. 89-114). Newbury Park, CA: Sage Publications.

Murphy, B. C. (1994). Difference and diversity: Gay and lesbian couples. *Social Services for Gay and Lesbian Couples, 1,* 5-31.

Muzio, C. (1999). Lesbian co-parenting: On being/being with the invisible (m)other. In J. Laird (Ed.), *Lesbians and lesbian families: Reflections on theory and practice* (pp. 197-211). New York: Columbia University Press.

Nakajima, G. A., Chan, Y. H., & Lee, K. (1996). Mental health issues for gay and lesbian Asian Americans. In R. P. Cabaj & T. S. Stein (Eds.), *Textbook of homosexuality and mental health* (pp. 563-581). Washington, DC: American Psychiatric Press.

Nakamura, K. (1997). Narrating ourselves: Duped or duplicitous? In B. Bullough, V. L. Bullough & J. Elias (Eds.), *Gender blending* (pp. 74-86). Amherst, NY: Prometheus Books.

Nakayama, T., & Corey, F. C. (1993). Homosexuality. In R. Kastenbaum (Ed.), *Encyclopedia of adult development* (pp. 208-215). Phoenix, AZ: Oryx.

Nardi, P. M. (1999). *Gay men's friendships: Invincible communities.* Chicago: University of Chicago Press.

National Coalition of Anti-Violence Programs. (2000). *Anti-lesbian, gay, transgender, and bisexual violence in 1999.* New York: New York City Gay and Lesbian Anti-Violence Project.

National Coalition of Anti-Violence Programs. (2004). Media release. Available online at <http://www.avp.org/publications/media/20040311_NCAVP_HateViolence.htm>.

National Gay and Lesbian Task Force Policy Institute. (2000). Seniors. Available online at <http://www.thetaskforce.org>.

Nations, L. (1997). Lesbian mothers: A descriptive study of a distinctive family structure. *Journal of Gay & Lesbian Social Services, 7,* 23-47.

Neisen, J. H. (1990). Heterosexism: Redefining homophobia for the 1990s. *Journal of Gay & Lesbian Psychotherapy, 1,* 21-35.

Nemoto, T., Luke, D., Mano, L., Ching, A., & Patria, J. (1999). HIV risk behaviors among male-to-female transgenders in comparison with homosexual or bisexual males and heterosexual females. *AIDS Care, 11,* 297-312.

Nestle, J. (1992). *The persistent desire: A femme-butch reader.* Boston: Alyson Press.

Nguyen, N. A. (1992). In L. A. Vargas & J. D. Koss-Chioino (Eds.), *Working with culture: Psychotherapeutic interventions with ethnic minority children and adolescents* (pp. 204-222). San Francisco, CA: Jossey-Bass.

Nichols, M. (1988). Bisexuality in women: Myths, realities, and implications for therapy. *Women and Therapy, 7,* 235-252.

Nichols, M. (1990). Lesbian relationships: Implications for the study of sexuality and gender. In D. P. McWhirter, S. A. Sanders, & J. M. Reinisch (Eds.), *Homosexuality/heterosexuality: Concepts of sexual orientation* (pp. 350-364). New York: Oxford University Press.

Nolo. (2004). Marriage rights and benefits. Available at <http://www.nolo.com/lawcenter/ency/article.cfm/ObjectID/E0366844-7992-4018-B581C6AE9BF8B045/catID/697DBAFE-20FF-467A-9E9395985EE7E825>.

Nurius, P. S. (1983). Mental health implications of sexual orientation. *Journal of Sex Research, 19,* 119-136.

Ochs, R. (Ed.). (2001). *The bisexual resource guide* (Fourth ed.). Boston: Bisexual Resource Center.

O'Connell, A. (1993). Voices from the heart: The developmental impact of a mother's lesbianism on her adolescent children. *Smith College Studies in Social Work, 63,* 281-299.

Oetjen, H., Rothblum, E. D. (2000). When lesbians aren't gay: Factors affecting depression among lesbians. *Journal of Homosexuality, 39,* 49-73.

Off Pink Collective. (1988). *Bisexual lives.* London: Off Pink Publishing.

Okun, B. F. (1996). *Understanding diverse families: What practitioners need to know.* New York: Guilford Press.

Olson, E. D., & King, C. A. (1995). Gay and lesbian self-identification: A response to Rotheram-Boras and Fernandez. *Suicide and Life-Threatening Behavior, 25,* 35-39.

Omoto, A., & Crain, A. (1995). AIDS volunteerism: Lesbian and gay community-based responses to HIV. In G. Herek & B. Greene (Eds.), *AIDS, identity and community: The HIV epidemic and lesbians and gay men* (pp. 187-209). Thousand Oaks, CA: Sage.

Original Prime Times Worldwide. (1998). *Who are prime timers?* Available online at <http://www.primetimers.org>.

Otis, M. D., & Skinner. W. F. (1996). The prevalence of victimization and its effect on mental well-being among lesbian and gay people. *Journal of Homosexuality, 30,* 3, 33-56.

Parks, C. (1999). Lesbian identity development: An examination of differences across generations. *American Journal of Orthopsychiatry, 69,* 347-361.

Partners Against Hate. (2003). 2002 FBI hate crimes statistics. Available online at <http://www.partnersagainsthate.org/law_enforcement/2003_fbi_facts.html>.

Patterson, C. J. (1992). Children of lesbian and gay men. *Journal of Sex Research, 30,* 62-69.

Patterson, C. J. (1994). Lesbian and gay families. *Current Directions in Psychological Science, 3,* 62-64.

Patterson, C. J. (1995). Lesbian mothers, gay fathers, and their children. In A. R. D'Augelli and C. J. Patterson (Eds.), *Lesbian, gay, and bisexual identities over the lifespan: Psychological perspectives* (pp. 262-290). Oxford: Oxford University Press.

Patterson, C., & Chan, R. (1997). Gay fathers. In M. E. Lamb (Ed.), *The role of father in child development* (pp. 245-260). New York: Wiley.

Patterson, D. G., & Schwartz, P. (1994). The social construction of conflict in intimate same-sex couples. In D. D. Cahn (Ed.), *Conflict in personal relationships* (pp. 3-26). Hillsdale, NJ: Lawrence Erlbaum.

Paul, J. P. (1988). Counseling issues in working with a bisexual population. In M. Shernoff & W. A. Scott (Eds.), *The sourcebook on lesbian/gay health care* (Second ed.) (pp. 142-150). Washington, DC: National Lesbian/Gay Health Foundation.

Paul, J. P. (1992). "Biphobia" and the construction of a bisexual identity. In M. Shernoff & W. A. Scott (Eds.), *The sourcebook on lesbian/gay health care* (Second ed.) (pp. 259-264). Washington, DC: National Lesbian/Gay Health Foundation.

Paul, J. P. (1996). Bisexuality: Exploring/exploding the boundaries. In R. C. Savin-Williams & K. M. Cohen (Eds.), *The lives of lesbian, gay men, and bisexuals: Children to adults* (pp. 436-461). Ft. Worth, TX: Harcourt Brace.

Paul, J. P., Hays, R. B., & Coates, T. J. (1995). The impact of the HIV epidemic on U.S. gay male communities. In A. R. D'Augelli & C. J. Patterson (Eds.), *Lesbians, gay, and bisexual identities over the lifespan: Psychological perspectives* (pp. 347-397). New York: Oxford.

Peplau, L. A. (1982-1983). Research on homosexual couples: An overview. *Journal of Homosexuality, 8,* 3-21.

Peplau, L. A. (1983a). Roles and gender. In H. H. Kelly, E. Berscheid, A. Christensen, J. H. Harvey, T. L. Huston, G. Levinger, E. McClintock, L. A. Peplau, & D. R. Peterson (Eds.), *Close relationships* (pp. 220-264). San Francisco: Freeman.

Peplau, L. A. (1983b). What homosexuals want. In O. Pocs (Ed.), *Human sexuality* (pp. 201-207). New York: Guilford Press.

Peplau, L. A. (1993). Lesbian and gay relationships. In L. D. Garnets and D. C. Kimmel (Eds.), *Psychological perspectives on lesbian and gay male experiences* (pp. 395-419). New York: Columbia University Press.

Peplau, L. A., & Amaro, H. (1982). Understanding lesbian relationships. In W. Paul, J. D. Weinrich, J. C. Gonsiorek, & M. E. Hotvedt (Eds.). *Homosexuality: Social, psychological, and biological issues* (pp. 233-248). Beverly Hills, CA: Sage Publications.

Peplau, L. A., & Cochran, S. D. (1990). A relational perspective on homosexuality. In D. P. McWhirter, S. A. Saunders, & J. M. Reinisch (Eds.), *Homosexuality/heterosexuality: Concepts of sexual orientation* (pp. 321-349). New York: Oxford University Press.

Plummer, K. (1995). *Telling sexual stories: Power, change and social worlds.* London: Routledge.

Ponse, B. (1980). Lesbians and their worlds. In J. Marmor (Ed.), *Homosexual behavior: A modern reappraisal* (pp. 157-175). New York: Basic Books.

Pope, M. (1995). The "salad bowl" is big enough for us all: An argument for the inclusion of lesbians and gay men in any definition of multiculturalism. *Journal of Counseling & Development, 73,* 301-304.

Pope, M. (1996). Gay and lesbian career counseling: Special career counseling issues. *Journal of Gay & Lesbian Social Services, 4,* 91-105.

Pope, M. (1997). Sexual issues for older lesbians and gays. *Topics in Geriatric Rehabilitation, 12,* 53-60.

Pope, M., & Schulz, R. (1990). Sexual attitudes and behavior in midlife and aging homosexual males. *Journal of Homosexuality, 20,* 169-177.

Pope, R. L., & Reynolds, A. L. (1991). Including bisexuality: It's more than just a label. In N. J. Evans & V. A. Walls (Eds.), *Beyond tolerance: Gays, lesbians and bisexuals on campus* (pp. 205-212). Alexandria, VA: American College Personnel Association.

Pride Senior Network (2001). *Pride Senior Network.* Available online at <www.pridesenior.org>.

Pusey, A. (2003, June 27). New day for gay Americans. *The Dallas Morning News*, p. 1A.

Quam, J. K. (1993). Gay and lesbian aging. *Siecus Report, 21*, 10-12.

Quam, J. K., & Whitford, G. S. (1992). Adaptation and age-related expectations of older gay and lesbian adults. *Gerontologist, 32*, 367-374.

Quittner, J. (2002, July 9). Where will they live? *The Advocate*, 22-23.

Radkowsky, M., & Siegel, L. J. (1997). The gay adolescent: Stressors, adaptations, and psychosocial interventions. *Clinical Psychology Review, 17*, 191-216.

Rangaswami, K. (1982). Difficulties in arousing and increasing heterosexual responsiveness in a homosexual: A case report. *Indian Journal of Clinical Psychology, 9*, 147-151.

Raphael, S., & Robinson, M. (1980). The older lesbian. *Alternative Lifestyles, 3*, 207-229.

Raphael, S., & Robinson, M. (1981). Lesbians and gay men in later life. *Generations, 6*, 16-18.

Raphael, S., & Robinson, M. (1984). The older lesbian: Love relationships and friendship patterns. In J. T. Darty & S. Potter (Eds.), *Women-identified women* (pp. 67-82). Palo Alto, CA: Mayfield.

Razzano, L. A., Matthews, A., & Hughes, T. L. (2002). Utilization of mental health services: A comparison of lesbian and heterosexual women. *Journal of Gay & Lesbian Social Services, 14*, 51-87.

Reid, J. D. (1995). Development in late life: Older lesbian and gay lives. In A. R. D'Augelli & C. J. Patterson (Eds.), *Lesbian, gay, and bisexual identities over the lifespan: Psychological perspectives* (pp. 215-240). New York: Oxford University Press.

Religious Tolerance.org (2004). Same-sex marriages (SSM) & civil unions. Available online at <http://www.religioustolerance.org/hom_marr.htm>.

Remafedi, G. (1987). Male homosexuality: The adolescent's perspective. *Pediatrics, 79*, 326-330.

Reuters (2004). Spain to approve gay marriage in 2 weeks. Available online at <http://www.reuters.co.us/newsPackageArticle.jhmtl?type=worldnews&storyID=586449&section=news>.

Reyes, M. (1992). Women's studies programs in Latin America: A source of empowerment. (Doctoral dissertation, University of Massachusetts, 1992). *Dissertation Abstracts International, 53* (6-A), 1819.

Ricketts, W., & Achtenberg, R. (1990). Adoption and foster parenting for lesbians and gay men: Creating new traditions in families. *Marriage & Family Review, 14*, 83-118.

Riddle, D. (1996). Riddle homophobia scale. In M. Adams, P. Brighham, P. Dalpes, & L. Marchesani (Eds.), *Social diversity and social justice: Gay, lesbian, and bisexual oppression* (p. 31). Dubuque, IA: Kendall/Hunt Publishing.

Ridge, D., Minichiello, V., & Plummer, D. (1997). Queer connections: Community, "the scene" and an epidemic. *Journal of Contemporary Ethnography, 26*, 146-181.

Roberts, P., & Newton, P. M. (1987). Levinsonian studies of women's adult development. *Psychology and Aging, 2,* 54-163.

Robinson, M. K. (1980). The older lesbian (Master's thesis, California State University, Dominguez Hills, 1979). *Masters Abstracts International, 18,* 135.

Robson, R. (1995). Our relationships and their laws. In K. Jay (Ed.), *Dyke life: From growing up to growing old, a celebration of the lesbian experience* (pp. 127-140). New York: Basic Books.

Rodriguez, F. I. (1996). Understanding Filipino male homosexuality: Implications for social services. *Journal of Gay & Lesbian Social Services, 5,* 93-113.

Rogers, S. M., & Turner, C. F. (1991). Male-male sexual contact in the U.S.A.: Findings from five sample surveys, 1970-1990. *Journal of Sex Research, 48,* 491-519.

Rohrbaugh, J. B. (1992). Lesbian families: Clinical issues and theoretical implications. *Professional Psychology: Research and Practice, 23,* 467-473.

Rosario, M., Meyer-Bahlburg, H. F. L., Hunter, J., Exner, T. M., Gwadz, M., & Keller, A. M. (1996). The psychosexual development of urban lesbian, gay, and bisexual youths. *Journal of Sex Research, 35,* 113-126.

Rose, S., & Zand, D. (2000). Lesbian dating and courtship from young adulthood to midlife. *Journal of Gay & Lesbian Social Services, 11,* 77-104.

Rosenberg, C. E., & Golden, J. (Eds.). (1992). *Framing disease: Studies in cultural history.* New Brunswick, NJ: Rutgers University Press.

Rosenfeld, C., & Emerson, S. (1998). A process model of supportive therapy for families of transgender individuals. In D. Denny (Ed.), *Current concepts of transgender identity* (pp. 391-400). New York: Garland.

Rosenfeld, D. (1999). Identity work among the homosexual elderly. *Journal of Aging Studies, 13,* 121-144.

Rosenfeld, D. (2003). *The changing of the guard: Lesbian and gay elders, and social change.* Philadelphia: Temple University Press.

Roth, S. (1985). Psychotherapy issues with lesbian couples. *Journal of Marital & Family Therapy, 11,* 273-286.

Rothberg, B., & Weinstein, D. L. (1996). A primer on lesbian and gay families. *Journal of Gay & Lesbian Social Services, 4,* 55-68.

Rothblum, E. D. (1994). Introduction to the special section: Mental health of lesbians and gay men. *Journal of Consulting and Clinical Psychology, 67,* 211-212.

Rothblum, E. D. (2000). Sexual orientation and sex in women's lives: Conceptual and methodological issues. *Journal of Social Issues, 56,* 193-204.

Rothblum, E. D., & Brehony, K. A. (1993). *Boston marriages: Romantic but asexual relationships among contemporary lesbians.* Amherst: University of Massachusetts Press.

Rothblum, E. D., Mintz, B., Cowan, D. B., & Haller, C. (1995). Lesbian baby boomers at midlife. In K. Jay (Ed.), *Dyke life: A celebration of the lesbian experience* (pp. 61-76). New York: Basic.

Rothschild, M. (1991). Life as improvisation. In B. Sang, J. Warshow, & A. Smith (Eds.), *Lesbians at midlife: The creative transition* (pp. 91-98). San Francisco: Spinsters.

Rupp, L. J. (1997). "Imagine my surprise": Women's relationships in historical perspective. *Journal of Lesbian Studies, 1,* 155-175.

Russell, G. M., & Bohan, J. S. (1999). Implications for clinical work. In J. S. Bohan & G. M. Russell (Eds.), *Conversations about psychology and sexual orientation* (pp. 31-56). New York: New York University Press.

Russo, A. J. (1982). Power and influence in the homosexual community: A study of three California cities (Doctoral dissertation). Claremont Graduate School. *Dissertation Abstracts International, 43,* 2B, 561.

Rust, P. C. (1993). "Coming out" in the age of social constructionism: Sexual identity formation among lesbian and bisexual women. *Gender & Society, 7,* 50-77.

Rust, P. C. (1995). *The challenge of bisexuality to lesbian politics: Sex, loyalty, and revolution.* New York: New York University Press.

Rust, P. C. (1996a). Finding a sexual identity and community: Therapeutic implications and cultural assumptions in scientific models of coming out. In E. D. Rothblum & L. A. Bond (Eds.), *Preventing heterosexism and homophobia* (pp. 87-123). Thousand Oaks, CA: Sage Publications.

Rust, P. C. (1996b). Monogamy and polyamory: Relationship issues for bisexuals. In B. A. Firestein (Ed.), *Bisexuality: The psychology and politics of an invisible minority* (pp. 127-148). Thousand Oaks, CA: Sage Publications.

Rutter, V., & Schwartz, P. (1996). Same-sex couples: Courtship, commitment, context. In A. W. Auhagen (Ed.), *The diversity of human relationships* (pp. 197-226). New York: Cambridge University Press.

Rutter, V., & Schwartz, P. (2000). Gender, marriage, and diverse possibilities for cross-sex and same-sex pairs. In D. H. Demo, K. R. Allen, & M. A. Fine (Eds.), *Handbook of family diversity* (pp. 59-81). New York: Oxford University Press.

Ryff, C. D. (1984). Personality development from the inside: The subjective experience of change in adulthood and aging. In P. P. Baltes & O. G. Brim (Eds.), *Life-span development and behavior, 6,* 243-279.

SAGE (2001). SAGE Web site. Available online at: <www.sageusa.org>.

Saghir, M. T., & Robbins, E. (1973). *Male and female homosexuality.* Baltimore: Williams and Wilkins.

Same-sex marriage ban passes (2004, September 3). *The Dallas Morning News,* p. 7A.

Sang, B. (1987, August). Existential issues of middle-aged lesbians. Paper presented at the annual convention of the American Psychological Association, New York.

Sang, B. (1990). Reflections of midlife lesbians on their adolescence. *Journal of Women & Aging, 2,* 111-117.

Sang, B. (1991). Moving toward balance and integration. In B. Sang, J. Warshow, & A. Smith (Eds.), *Lesbians at midlife: The creative transition* (pp. 206-214). San Francisco: Spinsters.

Sang, B. (1992a). Counseling and psychotherapy with midlife and older lesbians. In S. Dworkin & F. Gutiérrez (Eds.), *Counseling gay men and lesbians: Journey to the end of the rainbow* (pp. 35-48). Alexandria, VA: American Association for Counseling and Development.

Sang, B. (1992b). Psychotherapy with lesbians: Some observations and tentative generalizations. In W. R. Dynes (Ed.), *Encyclopedia of homosexuality* (pp. 260-269). New York: Garland.

Sang, B. (1993). Some existential issues of midlife lesbians. In L. D. Garnets & D. C. Kimmel (Eds.), *Psychological perspectives on lesbian and gay male experiences* (pp. 500-516). New York: Columbia University Press.

Savin-Williams, R. (1994). Verbal and physical abuse as stressors in the lives of lesbian, gay male, and bisexual youths: Associations with school problems, running away, substance abuse, prostitution, and suicide. *Journal of Consulting and Clinical Psychology, 62,* 260-269.

Savin-Williams, R. C. (1996). Ethnic-and sexual-minority youth. In R. C. Savin-Williams & K. M. Cohen (Eds.), *The lives of lesbian, gay men, and bisexuals: Children to adults* (pp. 152-165). Ft. Worth, TX: Harcourt Brace.

Savin-Williams, R. C. (1998a). *". . . and then I became gay": Young men's stories.* New York: Routledge.

Savin-Williams, R. C. (1998b). Lesbian, gay, and bisexual youths' relationships with their parents. In C. J. Patterson & A. R. D'Augelli (Eds.), *Lesbian, gay, and bisexual identities in families: Psychological perspectives* (pp. 75-98). New York: Oxford University Press.

Savin-Williams, R. C., & Diamond, L. M. (1999). Sexual orientation. In W. K. Silverman & T. H. Ollendick (Eds.), *Developmental issues in the clinical treatment of children* (pp. 241-258). Boston: Allyn & Bacon.

Savin-Williams, R. C., & Diamond, L. M. (2000). Sexual identity trajectories among sexual-minority youths: Gender comparisons. *Archives of Sexual Behavior, 29,* 607-627.

Scasta, D. (1998). Issues in helping people come out. *Journal of Gay and Lesbian Psychotherapy, 2,* 87-98.

Schatz, B., & K. O'Hanlan (1994). *Anti-gay discrimination in medicine: Results of a national survey of lesbian, gay and bisexual physicians.* San Francisco: American Association of Physicians for Human Rights.

Schneider, M. (2002, June 2). Floridian who came out of closet at 75 recounts decades-long journey. *The Dallas Morning News,* p. 10A.

Schope, R. D. (2002). The decision to tell: Factors influencing the disclosure of sexual orientation by gay men. *Journal of Gay & Lesbian Social Services, 14,* 1-21.

Schreurs, K. M. G., & Buunk, B. P. (1996). Closeness, autonomy, equity, and relationship satisfaction in lesbian couples. *Psychology of Women Quarterly, 20,* 577-592.

Schultz, G. (2001). Daughters of Bilitis: Literary genealogy and lesbian authenticity. *QLG: A Journal of Lesbian and Gay Studies, 7,* 377-389.

Scott, R. R., & Ortiz, E. T. (1996). Marriage and coming out: Four patterns in homosexual males. *Journal of Gay & Lesbian Social Services, 4,* 67-79.

Scrivner, R., & Eldridge, N. S. (1995). Lesbian and gay family psychology. In R. H. Mikesell, D. D. Lusterman, & S. H. McDaniel (Eds.), *Integrating family therapy: Handbook of family psychology and systems theory* (pp. 327-345). Washington, DC: American Psychological Association.

Sears, J. T. (1993/1994). Challenges for educators: Lesbian gay, and bisexual families. *High School Journal, 77,* 138-156.

Sears, J. T., & Williams, W. L. (Eds) (1997). *Overcoming heterosexism and homophobia: Strategies that work.* New York: Columbia University Press.

2nd Canada court backs gay marriage (2003, July 9). *The Dallas Morning News,* p. 9A.

Segal-Sklar, S. (1995). Lesbian parenting: Radical or retrograde? In K. Jay (Ed.), *Dyke life: A celebration of the lesbian experience* (pp. 174-191). New York: Basic Books.

Seidman, S. (2002). *Beyond the closet: The transformation of gay and lesbian life.* New York: Routledge.

Seil, D. (1996). Transsexuals: The boundaries of sexual identity and gender. In R. P. Cabaj & T. S. Stein (Eds.), *Textbook of homosexuality and mental health* (pp. 743-762). Washington, DC: American Psychiatric Press.

Sell, R. L. (1996). The Sell assessment of sexual orientation: Background and scoring. *Journal of Gay, Lesbian, and Bisexual Identity, 1,* 295-310.

Shankle, M. D., Maxwell, C. A., Katzman, E. S., & Landers, S. (2003). An invisible population: Older lesbian, gay, bisexual, and transgender individuals. *Clinical Research and Regulatory Affairs, 20,* 159-182.

Sharp, C. E. (1997). Lesbianism and later life in an Australian sample: How does development of one affect anticipation of the other? *Journal of Gay, Lesbian, and Bisexual Identity, 2,* 247-263.

Shenk, D. (1998). *Someone to lend a helping hand: Women growing old in rural America.* Newark, NJ: Gordon and Breach.

Shenk, D., & Fullmer, E. (1996). Significant relationships among older women: Cultural and personal constructions of lesbianism. *Journal of Women & Aging, 8,* 75-89.

Shernoff, M. (1996). Gay men choosing to be fathers. In M. Shernoff (Ed.), *Human services for gay people: Clinical and community practice* (pp. 41-54). Binghamton, NY: Harrington Park Press.

Shernoff, M. (1998). Getting started: Basic skills for effective social work with people with HIV and AIDS. In D. M. Aronstein & B. J. Thompson (Eds.), *HIV and social work: A practitioner's guide* (pp. 27-49). Binghamton, NY: The Harrington Park Press.

Shively, M. G., & De Cecco, J. P. (1977). Components of sexual identity. *Journal of Homosexuality, 3,* 41-48.

Shively, M. G., Jones, C., & De Cecco, J. (1983-1984). Research on sexual orientation: Definition and methods. *Journal of Homosexuality, 9,* 127-136.

Silberman, B., & Walton, R. (1986, March). Life satisfaction factors and older lesbians. Paper presented at the National Lesbian/Gay Health Conference, Washington, DC.

Silverstein, C. (1981). *Man to man: Gay couples in America.* New York: William Morrow.

Silverstein, C. (1991). Psychological and medical treatments of homosexuality. In J. C. Gonsiorek & J. D. Weinrich (Eds.), *Homosexuality: Research implications for public policy* (pp. 101-114). Newbury Park, CA: Sage Publications.

Silverstein, C. (1996). History of treatment. In R. P. Cabaj & T. S. Stein (Eds.), *Textbook of homosexuality and mental health* (pp. 3-16). Washington, DC: American Psychiatric Press.

Slusher, M., Mayer, C., & Dunkle, R. (1996). Gays and Lesbians Older and Wiser (GLOW): A support group for older gay people. *Gerontologist, 36,* 118-123.

Smith, A. (1997). Cultural diversity and the coming-out process: Implications for clinical practice. In B. Greene (Ed.), *Ethnic and cultural diversity among lesbians and gay men* (pp. 279-300). Thousand Oaks, CA: Sage Publications.

Smith, B. (Ed.). (1983). *Home girls: A black feminist anthology.* New York: Kitchen Table.

Smith, R. G., & Brown, R. A. (1998). The impact of social support on gay male couples. *Journal of Homosexuality, 33,* 39-61.

Solarz, A. L. (Ed.) (1999). *Lesbian health: Current assessment and directions for the future.* Washington, DC: National Academy Press, Institute of Medicine.

Sorensen, L., & Roberts, S. J. (1997). Lesbian uses of and satisfaction with mental health services: Results from Boston lesbian health project. *Journal of Homosexuality, 33,* 35-49.

Stall, R., & Catania, J. (1994). AIDS risk behaviors among late middle-aged and elderly Americans. *Archives of Internal Medicine, 154,* 57-63.

Stanley, J. L. (1996). The lesbian's experience of friendship. In J. S. Weinstock & E. D. Rothblum (Eds.), *Lesbian friendships: For ourselves and each other* (pp. 39-59). New York: New York University Press.

Stateline.org (2004). 50-state rundown on same-sex marriage laws. Available online at <http://www.stateline.org/stateline?pa=story&sa=showStoryInfo&id=353058&columns=true>.

Stein, E. (1999). *The mismeasure of desire: The science, theory, and ethics of sexual orientation.* New York: Oxford University Press.

Stein, G. L., & Bonuck, K. A. (2001). Attitudes of end-of-life care and advance care planning in the lesbian and gay community. *Journal of Palliative Medicine, 4,* 173-190.

Stein, M. (1983). *In midlife: A Jungian perspective.* Dallas: Spring.

Stein, T. S. (1993). Overview of new developments in understanding homosexuality. *Review of Psychiatry, 12,* 9-40.

Stevens, P. E. (1994). Lesbians' health-related experiences of care and non-care. *Western Journal of Nursing Research, 16,* 639-659.

Stiglitz, E. (1990). Caught between two worlds: The impact of a child on a lesbian couples relationship. *Women & Therapy, 10,* 99-116.

Stokes, J., & Damon, W. (1995). Counseling and psychotherapy for bisexual men. *Directions in Mental Health Counseling, 5,* 4-15.

Stokes, J. P., Miller, R. L., & Mundhenk, R. (1998). Toward an understanding of behaviorally bisexual men: The influence of context and culture. *Canadian Journal of Human Sexuality, 7,* 1-12.

Storms, M. D. (1980). Theories of sexual orientation. *Journal of Personality and Social Psychology, 38,* 783-792.

Strommen, E. F. (1989). "You're a what?" Family members' reactions to the disclosure of homosexuality. *Journal of Homosexuality, 18,* 37-58.

Strommen, E. F. (1990). Hidden branches and growing pains: Homosexuality and the family tree. *Marriage & Family Review, 14,* 9-34.

Sykes, D. L. (1999). Transgendered people: An invisible population. *California HIV/AIDS Update, 12,* 80-85.

Tasker, F. L., & Golombok, S. (1997). *Growing up in a lesbian family: Effects on child development.* New York: Guilford Press.

Tewksbury, R., & Gagné, G. (1996). Transgenderists: Products of non-normative intersections of sex, gender, and sexuality. *Journal of Men's Studies, 5,* 105-129.

Tewksbury, R., Grossi, E. L., Suresh, G., & Helms, J. (1999). Hate crimes against gay men and lesbian women: A routine activity approach for predicting victimization risk. *Humanity and Society, 23, 125-142.*

Thompson, C. A. (1992). Lesbian grief and loss issues in the coming-out process. *Women & Therapy, 12,* 175-185.

Thompson, N. L., McCandless, B. R., & Strickland, B. (1971). Personal adjustment of male and female homosexuals and heterosexuals. *Journal of Abnormal Psychology, 76,* 237-240.

Timberlake, E. M., & Cook, K. O. (1984). Social work and the Vietnamese refugee. *Social Work, 29,* 108-113.

Tofoya, T. N. (1996). Native two-spirit people. In R. P. Cabaj & T. S. Stein (Eds.), *Textbook of homosexuality and mental health* (pp. 603-617). Washington, DC: American Psychiatric Press.

Tofoya, T. N. (1997). Native gay and lesbian issues: The two-spirited. In B. Greene (Ed.), *Ethnic and cultural diversity among lesbians and gay men* (pp. 1-10). Thousand Oaks, CA: Sage Publications.

Trippet, S., & Bain, J. (1992). Reasons American lesbians fail to seek traditional health care. *Health Care for Women International Special Issue: Lesbian health: What are the issues? 13,* 145-153.

Tully, C. (1983). Social support systems of a selected sample of older women. Unpublished doctoral dissertation, Virginia Commonwealth University, Richmond.

Tully, C. (1988). Caregiving: What do midlife lesbians view as important? *Journal of Gay & Lesbian Psychotherapy, 1,* 87-103.

Tully, C. (2000). *Lesbians, gays, and the empowerment perspective.* New York: Columbia University Press.

Turner, P. H., Scadden, L., & Harris, M. B. (1990). Parenting in gay and lesbian families. *Journal of Gay & Lesbian Psychotherapy, 1,* 55-66.

Udis-Kessler, A. (1996). Challenging the stereotypes. In S. Rose & C. Stevens (Eds.), *Bisexual horizons: Politics, histories, lives* (pp. 45-57). London: Lawrence & Wisehart.

Uribe, V., & Harbeck, K. (1991). Coming out of the classroom closet. *Journal of Homosexuality, 22,* 9-27.

Vacha, K. (1985). *Quiet fire: Memoirs of older gay men.* Trumansburg, NY: Crossing Press.

Vaid, U. (1995). *Virtual equality: The mainstreaming of gay and lesbian liberation.* New York: Anchor Books.

Vaillant, G. (1977). *Adaptation to Life.* Boston: Little, Brown.

Vaillant, G. (1993). *The wisdom of the ego.* Cambridge, MA: Harvard University Press.

Van de Meide, W. (2000). *Legislating equality: A review of laws affecting gay, lesbian, bisexual, and transgendered people in the United States.* New York: Policy Institute of the National Gay and Lesbian Task Force.

Vargo, M. E. (1998). *Acts of disclosure: The coming-out process of contemporary gay men.* New York: Harrington Park Press.

Ven, P. Van de, Rodden, P., Crawford, J., and Kippax, S. (1997). A comparative demographic and sexual profile of older homosexually active men. *Journal of Sex Research, 34,* 349-360.

Vetri, D. (1998). Almost everything you always wanted to know about lesbians and gay men, their families, and the law. *Southern University Law Review, 26,* 1-68.

Vincke, J., Bolton, R., & Miller, M. (1997). Younger versus older gay men: Risks, pleasures, and dangers of anal sex. *AIDS Care, 9,* 217-225.

Von Schulthess, B. (1992). Violence in the streets: Anti-lesbian assault and harassment in San Francisco. In G. M. Herek & K. T. Berrill (Eds.), *Hate crimes: Confronting violence against lesbians and gay men* (pp. 65-75). Newbury Park, CA: Sage Publications.

Wahler, J., & Gabbay, S. G. (1997). Gay male aging: A review of the literature. *Journal of Gay & Lesbian Social Services, 6,* 1-20.

Waldo, C. R., Hesson-McInnis, M. S., & D'Augelli, A. R. (1998). Antecedents and consequences of victimization of lesbian, gay, and bisexual young people: A structural model comparing rural university and urban samples. *American Journal of Community Psychology, 26,* 307-334.

Walters, A. S., & Phillips, C. P. (1994). Hurdles: An activity for homosexuality education. *Journal of Sex Education and Therapy, 20,* 198-203.

Walters, K. L. (1997). Urban lesbian and gay American Indian identity: Implications for mental health service delivery. *Journal of Gay & Lesbian Social Services, 6,* 43-65.

Warshow, J. (1991). How lesbian identity affects the mother/daughter relationship. In B. Sang, J. Warshow, & A. J. Smith (Eds.), *Lesbians at midlife: The creative transition* (pp. 80-83). San Francisco: Spinsters.

Weber, J. C. (1996). Social class as a correlate of gender identity among lesbian women. *Sex Roles, 35,* 271-280.

Weeks, J. (1983). The problem of older homosexuals. In J. Hart, & D. Richardson (Eds.), *The theory and practice of homosexuality* (pp. 177-185). London: Routledge Kegan Paul.

Weinberg, G. (1972). *Society and the healthy homosexual.* New York: St. Martin's.

Weinberg, M. S. (1970a). Homosexual samples: Differences and similarities. *Journal of Sex Research, 6,* 312-325.

Weinberg, M. S. (1970b). The male homosexual: Age-related variations in social and psychological characteristics. *Social Problems, 17,* 527-538.

Weinberg, M. S., & Williams, C. J. (1974). *Male homosexuals: Their problems and adaptations.* New York: Oxford University.

Weinberg, M. S., Williams, C. J., & Pryor, D. W. (1994). *Dual attraction: Understanding bisexuality.* New York: Oxford University Press.

Weinberg, M. S., Williams, C. J., & Pryor, D. W. (1998). Becoming and being "bisexual." In E. J. Haeberle & R. Gindorf (Eds.), *Bisexualities: The ideology and practice of sexual contact with both men and women* (pp. 169-181). New York: Continuum.

Weinberg, M. S., Williams, C. J., & Pryor, D. W. (2001). Bisexuals at midlife: Commitment, salience, and identity. *Journal of Contemporary Ethnography, 30,* 180-208.

Weinstock, J. S. (2000). Lesbian friendships at midlife: Patterns and possibilities for the 21st century. *Journal of Gay & Lesbian Social Services, 11,* 1-32.

Weitz, R. (1989). Uncertainty and the lives of persons with AIDS. *Journal of Health and Social Behavior, 30,* 270-281.

Weston, K. (1991). *Families we choose: Lesbians, gays, kinship.* New York: Columbia University Press.

Weston, K. (1996). *Render me, gender me: Lesbians talk sex, class, color, nation, studmuffins . . .* New York: Columbia University Press.

White, J. C., & Dull, V. T. (1997). Health risk factors and health-seeking behavior in lesbians. *Journal of Women's Health, 6,* 103-112.

Whitford, G. S. (1997). Realities and hopes for older gay males. *Journal of Gay & Lesbian Social Services, 6,* 79-95.

Whitman, C. (1972/1992). A gay manifesto. In K. Jay and A. Young (Eds.), *Out of the closets: Voices of gay liberation,* (Second ed.) (pp. 330-342). New York: New York University Press.

Whitney, C. (1990). *Uncommon lives: Gay men and straight women.* New York: Plume.

Whittlin, W. (1983). Homosexuality and child custody: A psychiatric viewpoint. *Conciliation Courts Review, 21,* 77-79.

Willhoite, M. (2000). *Daddy's Roommate.* Los Angeles, CA: Alyson Wonderland.

Williams, E. & Donnelly, J. (2002). Older Americans and AIDS: Some guidelines for prevention. *Social Work, 47,* 105-111.

Williamson, D. S. (1998). An essay for practitioners: Disclosure is a family event. *Family Relations, 47,* 23-25.

Wojciechowski, C. (1998). Issues in caring for older lesbians. *Journal of Gerontological Nursing, 24,* 28-33.

Wolf, D. C. (1978, November). Close friendship patterns of older lesbians. Paper presented at 30th annual convention of the Gerontological Society of America, Dallas, TX.

Wolf, D. G. (1982). *Growing older: Lesbians and gay men.* Berkeley: University of California.

Wolfenden, J. (1963). *Reports of the committee on homosexual offenses and prostitution.* New York: Stein and Daly.

Wooden, W. S., Kawasaki, H., & Mayeda, R. (1983). Lifestyles and identity maintenance among gay Japanese-American males. *Alternate Lifestyles, 5,* 236-243.

Woodman, N. J. (1987, September). Lesbian women in their midyears: Issues and implications for practice. Paper presented at the health/mental health conference of the National Association of Social Workers, New Orleans, LA.

Woolf, L. M. (2002). Gay and lesbian aging. *Siecus Report, 30,* 16-21.

Woolf, P. F. (1998). Mid-life transition to lesbian: Expanding consciousness of women. *Anthropology of Consciousness, 9,* 49-72.

Wyers, N. L. (1987). Homosexuality in the family: Lesbian and gay spouses. *Social Work, 32,* 143-148.

Yang, A. (1999) *From wrongs to rights: 1973-1999: Public opinion on gay and lesbian American moves toward equality.* Washington, DC: National Gay and Lesbian Task Force.

Yarhouse, M. A. (1999). Social cognition research on the formation and maintenance of stereotypes: Applications to marriage and family therapists working with homosexual clients. *American Journal of Family Therapy, 27,* 149-161.

Zinik, G. (1985). Identity conflict or adaptive flexibility? Bisexuality reconsidered. *Journal of Homosexuality, 11,* 7-19.

Zook, M. (2001). *Psychotherapy experiences of women attracted to both men and women.* San Francisco: California Institute of Integral Studies.

Zuger, B. (1984). Early effeminate behavior in boys: Outcome and significance for homosexuality. *Journal of Nervous and Mental Disorders, 172,* 90-97.

Index

Order a copy of this book with this form or online at:
http://www.haworthpress.com/store/product.asp?sku=5289

MIDLIFE AND OLDER LGBT ADULTS
Knowledge and Affirmative Practice for the Social Services

_____ in hardbound at $39.95 (ISBN: 0-7890-1835-7)

_____ in softbound at $24.95 (ISBN: 0-7890-1836-5)

Or order online and use special offer code HEC25 in the shopping cart.

COST OF BOOKS_____

POSTAGE & HANDLING_____
(US: $4.00 for first book & $1.50
for each additional book)
(Outside US: $5.00 for first book
& $2.00 for each additional book)

SUBTOTAL_____

IN CANADA: ADD 7% GST_____

STATE TAX_____
(NJ, NY, OH, MN, CA, IL, IN, PA, & SD
residents, add appropriate local sales tax)

FINAL TOTAL_____
(If paying in Canadian funds,
convert using the current
exchange rate, UNESCO
coupons welcome)

☐ **BILL ME LATER:** (Bill-me option is good on US/Canada/Mexico orders only; not good to jobbers, wholesalers, or subscription agencies.)
☐ Check here if billing address is different from shipping address and attach purchase order and billing address information.

Signature_____

☐ **PAYMENT ENCLOSED: $**_____

☐ **PLEASE CHARGE TO MY CREDIT CARD.**

☐ Visa ☐ MasterCard ☐ AmEx ☐ Discover
☐ Diner's Club ☐ Eurocard ☐ JCB

Account # _____

Exp. Date_____

Signature_____

Prices in US dollars and subject to change without notice.

NAME_____
INSTITUTION_____
ADDRESS_____
CITY_____
STATE/ZIP_____
COUNTRY_____ COUNTY (NY residents only)_____
TEL_____ FAX_____
E-MAIL_____

May we use your e-mail address for confirmations and other types of information? ☐ Yes ☐ No
We appreciate receiving your e-mail address and fax number. Haworth would like to e-mail or fax special discount offers to you, as a preferred customer. **We will never share, rent, or exchange your e-mail address or fax number.** We regard such actions as an invasion of your privacy.

Order From Your Local Bookstore or Directly From
The Haworth Press, Inc.

10 Alice Street, Binghamton, New York 13904-1580 • USA
TELEPHONE: 1-800-HAWORTH (1-800-429-6784) / Outside US/Canada: (607) 722-5857
FAX: 1-800-895-0582 / Outside US/Canada: (607) 771-0012
E-mailto: orders@haworthpress.com

For orders outside US and Canada, you may wish to order through your local
sales representative, distributor, or bookseller.
For information, see http://haworthpress.com/distributors

(Discounts are available for individual orders in US and Canada only, not booksellers/distributors.)

PLEASE PHOTOCOPY THIS FORM FOR YOUR PERSONAL USE.
http://www.HaworthPress.com   BOF04